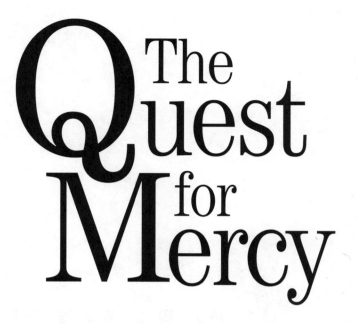

The Quest for Mercy

The forgotten ingredient in health care reform

The Quest for Mercy

The forgotten ingredient in health care reform

By Roger J. Bulger, M.D.

CARDEN JENNINGS
PUBLISHING CO., LTD.

ISBN 1-891524-01-1

Carden Jennings Publishing Co., Ltd.
The Blake Center, Suite 200
1224 West Main Street
Charlottesville, VA 22903
U.S.A.

Copies of this book may be purchased from: Carden Jennings Publishing Co., Ltd., The Blake Center, Suite 200, 1224 West Main St., Charlottesville, VA 22903; Phone: 804/979-4913; Fax: 804/979-4025. Price: $10.00 (U.S.)

T his book is dedicated to the memory of Matthew Warpick, MD, and other caregivers like him. Dr. Warpick was a physician in New York City who served generations of residents of a west Harlem neighborhood for sixty-seven years. He healed, counseled, and listened to his patients; in return, he accepted whatever they could pay. Dr. Warpick finally closed his office when violence engulfed his neighborhood and he feared for the safety of two employees. At ninety-three years old and determined to stick by his patients, whom he considered his friends, Dr. Warpick replaced the living room furniture in his apartment with an examining table and some other medical equipment, planning to see patients six days a week. "People are losing faith in doctors and medicine," he explained, "and something must be done." He believed that without ready access to friendly, caring, science-based physicians, more and more people turn to nonscience-based alternative venues in their search for caring healers. Dr. Warpick's dedication surely changed the lives of his patients. His story, as reported by D. Gonzales in the New York Times, should motivate us all, whether entering or practicing scientific medicine, to try to do the same. Dr. Warpick saw patients into his ninety-sixth year. He died in January 1997.

Contents

Preface

This book is about medicine and the caregiver in today's society. I have written it from the perspective of an educator deeply involved in practicing and teaching medicine for almost thirty-five years. At first, I had only younger and future colleagues in mind. As the book progressed, however, I also attempted to make it a work of interest to anyone concerned with his or her own health in particular and with health care reform in general.

Health care is a wonderful calling because it involves the professional in all aspects at both extremes and along the full continuum of life's experiences. But on occasion over the years, I have found myself in circumstances demanding actions that have challenged the boundaries between my various life roles (physician, husband, father, son, brother, citizen, friend). The appropriate responses, however, were not articulated in medical textbooks. I wish that, as a medical student and young physician, I had been provoked to ponder some of the less concrete and less technical aspects of physicianhood—for example, dealing with the joy, birth, healing, growth, suffering, pain, separation, and death that I discuss in the following pages. They are compelling but often overlooked aspects of clinical practice that arise in one form or another every day.

During the course of writing this book, I suddenly found myself cast in yet another role. This time I was a patient. Furthermore, I was a patient with a complex, serious disease. My perspective on our health care system changed dramatically.

Health care reform is creating a complete turnaround in the financial incentives available to caregivers: previously paid for each intervention they performed, many are now paid to minimize their interventions or not intervene at all. As a result, the primary objective for many caregivers today may be cost containment. Does this mean that the growing prospective payment, capitated care system will so alter provider payment mechanisms that the core financial incentives for caregiving will become completely reversed?

Furthermore, because recent health care reform is also largely changing the method of rationing professional time, those caregivers whose time is excessively restricted may well lose altogether the time it takes to develop the trust that, in turn, empowers patients to enter into their own healing.

I believe my recent experience was highly positive, in part, because I never questioned the motivations of my caregivers, never worried that they had incentives to keep valuable treatments from me even when the prospects of full recovery were unclear. Thus I feel certain that we must find a way to restrain clinical costs without twisting the caregiver's motivation to help the patient or driving a wedge between the sufferer and the healer.

There is an order to the sequencing of the subjects I discuss in the following pages. The left side of my brain can argue that this ordering is rational, with each chapter flowing from the preceding chapter until the story emerges of what it takes to make a full-blown healer. In all honesty, however, I can only say that the chapters represent pieces to a puzzle that, if put together in any order through an individual's educational life experiences, represent the essentials of the mature, twenty-first century scientific healer, no matter how or when the essentials are acquired.

I use the term "scientific healer" to recognize that there are other "healers" out there who seem capable of eliciting a suffering person's own healing powers. Modern medicine, however, empowers its practitioners with many enormously effective scientific interventions that, if grafted onto the elements of being a healing person, open up extraordinary capacities to benefit people.

I start with the difference between illness, disease, and suffering; the peculiarly American slant that we bring to the condition of suffering; and some first-hand experiences of physicians as patients (including myself) in section I.

Because understanding and easing the suffering of a patient can eventually be only as effective as the caregiver's communication skills, section II discusses these skills, which form the basis of a trusting relationship with the patient and also facilitate the patient's self-healing capacities. The second section also examines the essentials of the Hippocratic oath, the placebo effect, and some literature relating to self-healing. Seldom are therapeutic victories complete, however, and the true healer understands this fact of life almost instinctively. Thus, I also point out that whereas a return to full health can happen in one patient, perhaps the best outcome in the next patient leaves chronic debility or permanent loss. Just as this patient now needs to cope with a new reality, the caregiver must be certain the patient is not abandoned.

Section III deals with the tensions among the new, growing population-based emphasis on health status, health promotion, and disease prevention; the reductionist, biomolecular, disease-oriented paradigm that rules among most medical school faculty today; and the biopsychosocial paradigm, which takes the patient's feelings into account and seeks to bring the behavioral sciences to the relationship between patient and clinician.

In section IV, I explore the traditional relationship between patient and healer, and the new conflicts of interest and ethics that caregiving health professionals are beginning to face in these rapidly changing times. A revision of the Hippocratic oath is suggested that better mirrors the world in which tomorrow's caregivers will be rendering care. By analogy and extension, we come to the concept and characteristics of a therapeutic team of health professionals. (Today, of course, this health care team includes the patient.)

Note that almost all of my generalizations about the individual clinician refer to whatever collection of people and entities become part of what I call an "organized healing delivery system." But however we conceive of or refer to the way we provide health care in America, the next century must see us, the caregivers, improve both our individual and our collective performances as therapeutic agents. Only in this way can we bring humanity into our ever-increasingly technology-dominated enterprise.

Health care is a career that can marry marvelously the worlds of action, emotion, and mind. It remains one of the most rewarding careers available. Little more can be asked of a professional life. I hope this book makes the reader aware of the extraordinary breadth of interest and scholarship open to thinking caregivers who keep learning from a wide array of disciplines. I also trust that caregivers, policymakers, and the general public—potential patients all—will find food for thought in the following pages as America reflects on a health care system in flux.

Acknowledgments

Because my primary concern in this book is to communicate effectively with younger people, during the writing process I enlisted the aid of three people still in their third decade of life. The first was my daughter, Grace Bulger, who is an expert on the art of communication. After reviewing my previous writings in this area and some of the relevant medical literature, she prepared an initial draft of the chapter on communication and the arts in medicine. Elizabeth Bobby spent several months working with me before beginning her education to become a nurse practitioner. She helped with the whole manuscript, but was especially involved in the evolution of the chapters in Section I. Kara Reinhardt, while an undergraduate at Princeton University, helped by giving the completed manuscript a careful reading. Her opinions and reactions led me to make a number of substantive improvements, some of them quite major.

More recently, Denise Holmes, who has become a colleague, has lent her keen intellect, insight, and editorial skills to the effort. Many thanks also go to Richard Fletcher for his design and production expertise, and to Shirley Sirota Rosenberg for her assistance in the entire editing process.

My deepest thanks also must go to my personal physicians, Bryan Arling and Bruce Kessel, who have taken care of me and helped me to do my share in addressing my illness.

My personal thanks go to the McGovern Foundation for its ongoing support of my writing efforts over the past decade. Jack McGovern has been a true friend and benefactor for over twenty years, and it is unlikely that this book would have become a reality without his interest.

Last, I must mention several colleagues who read the complete manuscript at one stage or another, and who were kind enough to offer suggestions and encouragement. I cannot blame the deficiencies on them, but readily admit that their input was vital to the shape, organization, and content of the final product. They are Ruth Bulger, Jack Colwill, Ralph Crawshaw, Rich De Vaul, Leon Eisenberg, Elaine Larson, Sam Nixon, Marian Osterweis, Ed Pellegrino, Stan Reiser, David Rogers, John Stoeckle, Eleanor Sullivan, and Larry Tancredi.

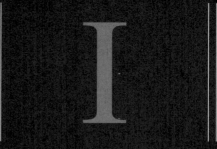

I

Why
Patients
Need
Healers

Chapter One

Understanding Illness, Disease, and Suffering

We spend much of our lives trying to avoid, ignore, or minimize suffering—but sooner or later it finds all of us. Suffering is part of the human condition. Caregivers, especially doctors and nurses, have a dramatically larger experience with suffering than others because they minister to those suffering people we call patients, a word that connotes suffering or endurance. In fact, I believe that you are not a patient if you are not suffering, and you cannot be an effective caregiver if you do not know a great deal about suffering and its alleviation.

The Connection and the Distinction

How do disease and illness connect to the concept of suffering? Simply put, disease plus suffering equals illness! There is a rich distinction between the two terms, disease and illness. A disease can be labeled (for example, diabetes, multiple sclerosis, tuberculosis, or breast cancer). The label typically refers to an identifiable pathologic state with a known or unknown cause, a pattern of symptomatic involvement and diagnostic laboratory tests, a describable clinical course, and a range of known courses that has been established by following the lives of previous patients. In each case, the hope is that a physiologically or molecularly precise, effective, and safe treatment will be discovered and made widely available.

Beyond Physical Pain

Illness, on the other hand, describes how that disease affects a particular patient because of that patient's life experiences, including the patient's ethnicity, age, sex, family, and sociocultural situation. The person's underlying emotional state and emotional response to the disease have a great influence on the illness. Understanding an individual's illness is essential to estimating the degree of suffering the patient is experiencing and, in turn, to establishing a method for helping the sufferer deal with the illness.

Fear of Death

Let me provide a simple example. From my own experience as an intern and resident, I concluded early on that virtually every patient who entered the hospital must be worrying about the increased possibility of dying, either from the disease, or the treatment, or the errors inherent in the health care system. Thus, while focusing on a particular disease, I found it extremely useful to anticipate these broader fears, recognizing and discussing them with the patient. The patients, I believe, were much happier and more confident in me because I foresaw and empathized with their concerns; they experienced less fear and anxiety from the hospitalization than otherwise would have been the case.

Because the disease/treatment environment can add to either the patient's illness burden or relief, caregivers need to anticipate all the forces affecting the patient's life and try to alleviate as many negative ones as possible. The most effective physicians are those who can combine their science-based competencies at diagnosing and treating disease with the capacity to join with the patient in combating the broader issues of illness and suffering.

Loss of Control

Although there are many different notions of suffering, there is an unusually strong convergence about the ultimate meaning of suffering. Eric Cassell, a physician, articulates this generally held meaning best when he describes suffering as a state of distress induced by the loss, or threatened loss, of control or meaning in one's life, or by the perceived disintegration of one's persona. Suffering, he asserts, is a feeling that goes beyond and is distinct from pain. Two persons may be exposed to the same pain, but suffer to different degrees. Suffering may also occur in the absence of pain, as in the anticipation of future pain. Cassell emphasizes the social and psychological foundations of suffering: "Suffering is a consequence of personhood—bodies do not suffer, persons do."

Dread of Abandonment

John Fortunato, in his recent discussion of the spiritual dilemma that the AIDS epidemic has forced upon society, underscores the idea of the sufferer being excluded, or feeling isolated, from society. He describes how an individual's suffering heightens when societal support systems seem to wither away as death becomes inevitable. Pediatrician R. Vieth also deals with these ideas in terms of their theological implications; I include such theological considerations in this discussion because many people in our society are influenced by them.

My own experience with a severely psychotic patient, whom I met when I was a fourth-year medical student, showed me how isolation itself can cause suffering. The patient rambled unintelligibly and people thought that she was hallucinating, a situation that hindered human interaction and increased this woman's isolation. As I came to know her, and explain more fully in chapter 4, I came to understand her vision of herself as an abandoned princess; in turn, my understanding helped to end her isolation and begin the long journey toward improving her health.

Anthropologist Margaret Mead has also equated suffering with exclusion from society, concluding that to reduce suffering as well as to increase the strength of society, all suffering citizens must be included in the fabric of society. Implicit in this argument is the assumption that a strong society takes care of its weakest members. As the poet William Blake wrote, "The dog starv'd at his master's gate/Predicts the ruin of the state."

Loss of Esteem

Suffering seems infinite when self-respect is destroyed, suggests physician Howard Brody in *Stories of Sickness*. Conversely, suffering can be minimized if self-respect is maintained. In the context of these interweaving ideas, it is perhaps easier to understand how suffering accompanies grief, anxiety, depression, and other situations in which patients feel a high degree of personal inadequacy. This is why suffering strikes us all and is a universal characteristic of human life.

The suffering of Donald "Dax" Cowart, a young man recently out of the military, presents a compelling story, replete with lessons for future health professionals. As discussed by William May, an ethicist and physician, in *The Patient's Ordeal*, this young man, severely burned in a propane gas explosion, asked the first passerby to get him a gun so that he could end his own life. He asked the rescue squad not to take him to the hospital, and he subsequently asked the emergency room staff not to treat him. He pleaded with anyone who would listen, "Please let me die."

Dax had suffered severe burns over two-thirds of his body, including third-degree burns to his face and hands and severe damage to his eyes. Even after the initial emergency treatment, Dax's prognosis for survival remained poor. Costly, painful, extensive burn therapy continued, however, even as Dax consistently demanded that treatment be discontinued and stated repeatedly over many months of treatment that he wanted to die.

In the story of a burn patient's painful rehabilitation, Dax's story amply illustrates profound suffering. Yet May explains how Dax's suffering was far broader than simply the physical pain of his burns:

> Short of suffering brain damage, perhaps no patient undergoes the massive alteration in self-perception and prospects that the burn victim must fear. And yet, even the burn victim and victims of other, lesser catastrophes do not suffer a total wipeout. The image of the Phoenix, risen from the ashes, partly misleads us, because the Phoenix remembers nothing of its former life. The burn victim, however, remembers his past. The persistence of memory both establishes continuity with his past but also reinforces his sense of distance from it. He remembers what he has lost and therefore grieves more deeply.

Dax's physical trauma was magnified by psychic suffering caused by the health care professionals' refusal to accede to his relentless demands. The emergency room staff assumed that he was not competent to refuse treatment and dismissed his plea as the typical reaction of a burn victim in pain. Many months later, a psychiatric evaluation found him to be competent, yet treatment continued.

May comments on how the professional's paternalistic approach clashes with the patient's autonomy:

> The provider has seen too many post-trauma depressives who have demanded that physicians stop treating them and then changed their minds later. But this suspicion of post-traumatic depressives discredits the patient's wishes and casts a long shadow into the future, particularly when the patient's opposition to a procedure seems to prove the patient's impaired capacity. The burden of proof thus effectively shifts from the physician having to justify his paternalistic intervention to the patient having to prove his competence.

Thus, the patient's physical suffering, grief, altered self-perception, depression, and anxiety about an uncertain future may be compounded by a caregiver's disregard for the patient's expressed preferences.

Dax survived, pursued his education, and among other activities has remained outspoken about the conflicts inherent in his situation. As I understand it, he is happy with the life he has made since his accident, but he remains adamant that he should have been allowed to die.

Chapter Two

The American Way of Suffering

A definitive analysis of our society's relationship to suffering is too complex to attempt in this short treatise. However, exploring some of the ways in which Americans may be insensitive to suffering, promote suffering, or fail to ameliorate suffering may help us reach a better understanding of American society's complex relationship with it. Because each of us is, to a significant degree, a product of our society, all aspiring health caregivers should give some thought to these matters. The study of suffering, strange as it may seem, is central to our education as caring health professionals.

Traditional Values

Life, liberty, the pursuit of happiness, individuality, and self-sufficiency: these are among the most fundamental of American values. Most people who have come to America left their own countries because they were poor, persecuted, or desperately unhappy with their governments. We are a nation with an inherent historical distrust of collectivity, especially as it is reflected in the federal government. We have had generations of success escaping initial poverty and getting out of the ghetto (although those possibilities seem to be decreasing). We have seen the progressive enhancement of our standard of living, first through westward expansion to our frontiers and then through the industrial revolution and into the postin-

dustrial era. We believe in the benefits of individual efforts to better oneself.*
We also believe that each of us should have as many years as possible to enjoy
life, liberty, and the pursuit of happiness. In fact, focusing on suffering might
almost be considered unpatriotic; after all, our Declaration of Independence
tells us to pursue happiness. Why dwell on suffering? Better to forestall, delay,
or deny it completely.

Individualism and Self-Determination

America's commitment to the individual is reflected in our health care organization and expenditure and, most clearly, in our love for the most dramatic of inno-
vations—even if aimed at saving just one life. Our nation is capable of spending
millions of dollars and riveting its collective attention for weeks on efforts to
recover a child who has fallen into a well or to rescue a person lost at sea. To save
a single premature infant in neonatal intensive care, we routinely spend substantial sums that could finance, if redirected, prenatal care for a large number of poor
women, thereby reducing the incidences of prematurity. Psychologist Arthur
Kleinman suggests that

> [P]erhaps North American culture's ideology of personal freedom and the pursuit of
> happiness has come to mean for many guaranteed freedom from the suffering of pain.
> This meaning clashes strikingly with the expectation in much of the non-industrialized
> world that pain is an expectable component of living and must be endured in silence.

Ben Franklin's *Poor Richard's Almanac* epitomizes Americans' reverence for individualism. "God helps those who help themselves," he wrote. Americans have
taken these words to heart. In 1835, Tocqueville worried about the implications
for Americans of their rampant individualism, which he saw manifested in a
growing number of American frontiersmen. These men had no need for community—they believed that with their family, their gun, and their good sense and
industry they could handle the world. Social scientists Robert Bellah and colleagues, in their analysis of 1980s America, hold that Tocqueville's concerns were
prophetic. Eric Cassell agrees: "The concentration on individuality by Western
culture for these last centuries . . . has obscured the more basic truth that we live
in a sea of others without whom existence is literally unthinkable."

---

*This belief, unfortunately, can also spawn the corollary perception that people who are in the midst of unfor-
tunate circumstances either brought their problems upon themselves or are too lazy to extract themselves
from their quandary.

Quest for Efficiency

Organization, linear behavior, and efficiency are integral features of the American work ethic and American success in the modern era. We work hard, move from one place to another often, and sacrifice much in the name of greater efficiency, greater productivity, and greater profits. When a family member dies, we tend to limit the mourning period to one or two days and then return to work to minimize the inconvenience to our coworkers and shelve our emotions. Grieving, after all, is not productive; moreover, it disrupts the equilibrium of a finely tuned corporate system. In this context, prolonged suffering appears to thrust an unseemly burden upon others; distancing or isolating ourselves from the normal environment may seem to be the most considerate act when we are bereaved people.

The Fighting Spirit

Americans admire fighters—take, for instance, John Wayne, Clint Eastwood, Michael Jordan, Scott O'Grady, Martina Navratilova, and even Rambo. Many of our friends, relatives, ancestors, and heroes fought their way out of poverty, ignorance, and hardship to attain better lives. Many of us may feel that God not only helps those who help themselves, but that God loves a fighter. At some level, we may, therefore, believe that people who do not fight their diseases are losers. Even children with cancer are frequently taught that defeating the disease depends on their healthy cells getting good and mad at the cancer cells. And, because a good fighter is supposed to fear nothing, we tend to hide the difficult issues posed by suffering and the concomitant fear of personal dissolution, focusing instead on the notion of bravery. Furthermore, and perhaps most destructively, when suffering cannot be avoided and death seems inevitable, sufferers may feel a sense of failure in their efforts to ward off the disease.

Dwindling Social Ties

Our ties to the traditional societal institutions—churches, clubs, hometowns, and families—that once provided structure and support to individuals have sustained much damage in America over the last fifty years. As the sense of community diminishes, a cultural emphasis on personal privacy, individual rights, and freedoms rises. In guarding this shared sense of individuality, we seem to pay less attention to those other, more community-oriented, beliefs and values that we share.

Our voting behavior and our approach to politics have become focused on selfish desires, small groups or subsets of society, and special interests. Unfortunately, this inwardness serves to further undermine community; the larger the number of factions, the smaller the number of groups who can achieve their goals. A case in point is the health care reform legislative debacle of 1994, in which a wide array of special interests thwarted the will of a large majority of citizens.

If suffering is a sort of separation that may be relieved by reincorporating with the group, the disintegration of social ties that link individuals to communities can only tend to make our culture increasingly unresponsive and insensitive to suffering in general. Thus, suffering gets interpreted as an individual problem, leading to an isolation that only serves to exacerbate the suffering. This seclusion, notes Eric Cassell, can further disrupt those aspects of personhood that require social contact: "Otherness is implied by self, and many, by one." As recognized by proponents of Twelve-Step programs and other group-centered therapies, sharing fears, feelings, and experiences can be a powerful tool for combating suffering.

Suffering as Punishment

Many Americans believe at some level that suffering is a proper punishment for sin and that the sufferer deserves to be shunned and to lose dignity in front of the rest of society. Religious belief systems sometimes contribute to this view; issues of suffering and pain are often entwined with the concept of evil in religious explanations of God's nature and intentions. Some religions teach that we deserve our suffering—that we suffer for Original Sin as well as for individual transgressions. Many religions also suggest that the evil or sin that precipitated the suffering is contagious.

Such beliefs have important implications for the sufferer. Elizabeth Heitman, who teaches in a program on humanities and technology in health care, notes that when suffering is interpreted as divine punishment, its association with evil may prompt others to reject the sufferer as contaminated. She writes, "Where suffering is interpreted as punishment, a necessary lesson, or an inevitable consequence of nature, the intervention of outsiders may be rejected as interference with the mechanisms of cosmic justice." This action, or, rather, inaction, serves to further isolate the sufferer, who has many other reasons to feel separated.

Patients whose afflictions are the result of such socially unacceptable practices as drunk driving, drug abuse, and sexual promiscuity may be more likely than other patients to have their suffering disregarded. This tendency on the part of caregivers may be especially true in settings where there are other suffering patients needing attention. It is far easier for a caregiver to feel empathy for a patient whose illness is unavoidable than for a patient who returns time and again for relief from a behaviorally induced disease.

Mass Media and Desensitization

Movies, news, and television drama series are so full of violence and death that it is rare to turn on the television without seeing or hearing about some horribly traumatic event. Explicit movies, for example, graphically illustrate how to kill, injure, or mutilate others or oneself, and the media make major figures of many of the sorriest examples of human degradation. The media not only feature violence; they tend to focus on the mundane, the material, the quick-fix, and the one-time around, thereby leaving unaddressed the suffering lurking in the background. Moreover, when suffering is portrayed on film, it is usually short-lived and often resolved in a fortunate turn of events. This casualness toward killing and death makes it easier and easier for society to minimize respect for life and more difficult to empathize with others who are suffering. We become desensitized.

Another way in which the media affect our relationship to suffering is through their love of wealth, fame, youth, beauty, and perfection. In the media, suffering, pain, and adjustment to adversity often seem alien to the American recipe for the good life.*

Desensitization to suffering also can occur in the health care setting. Urban, often overloaded emergency rooms are places where suffering is so common, it is no longer as appalling to the health care professionals as to persons not regularly exposed to such situations. Caregivers in general, regardless of their work setting, may be more desensitized to suffering than the general population, simply because they work daily amidst suffering. This circumstance highlights the tension inherent in a situation in which the importance of being efficient, objective, and analytical (and, in a sense, dispassionate) vies with the importance of recognizing suffering and showing compassion to those who suffer.

---

*This is not to say that the arts do not offer psychologically constructive and socially useful depictions of the true nature of suffering. As Aristotle believed, public presentations of tragedies can serve an important therapeutic function because of the emotional catharsis they engender in the audience.

Reductionist View of Medicine

The Newtonian, reductionist, biomolecular orientation of modern physician-hood emphasizes scientific intervention through emphasis on the molecular causes of, and therapies for, human disease. As a consequence, this view has little to do with such concepts as the healing relationship. According to Donald Seldin, one of the great figures in modern medicine who described this view some years ago, the needs and opportunities for molecular medicine are so great that physicians should focus their energies on the pursuit of diseases in terms of their molecular causes and therapies, leaving the psyches and personalities, wants and needs, hopes and fears, social problems, and familial relationships of patients in the domain of nurses and social workers. Kleinman perceives this orientation as somewhat built into this country's view of illness:

> Social reality is so organized that we do not routinely inquire into the meanings of illness any more than we regularly analyze the structure of our social world. Indeed, the everyday priority structure of medical training and of health care delivery, with its radically materialistic pursuit of the biological mechanism of disease, precludes such inquiry. It turns the gaze of the clinician, along with the attention of patients and families, away from decoding the salient meanings of illness for them, which interferes with recognition of disturbing but potentially treatable problems in their life world. The biomedical system replaces this allegedly "soft," therefore devalued, psychosocial concern with meanings with the scientifically "hard," therefore overvalued, technical quest for the control of symptoms. This pernicious value transformation is a serious failing of modern medicine: it disables the healer and disempowers the chronically ill.

Kleinman thus illuminates the important distinction between a disease, which can be diagnosed and treated at the molecular level, and the associated illness, which affects the whole of the patient's life and requires a broader perspective if therapeutic support is to be forthcoming.

If suffering is, in fact, a sense of impending personal disintegration, then clearly the reductionist physician described by Seldin is not predisposed to relieving emotional suffering and is likely not concerned with understanding or even recognizing suffering. Kleinman's view of the "technical quest for control of symptoms" points to a similar situation. In examining the Dax case, May noted that burn patients receive acute and follow-up treatment for their physical wounds, but that our society must invest more in rehabilitative and long-term care. The bottom-line message to patients and to society is one of excluding suffering from the purview of the high priests of modern medicine, those to whom we have given the vestments associated with marrying high technology with humanity. For the most part, suffering—that is, social and psychological pain—is not part of the healing equation.

Some Things We Can Do

So far in this discussion, I have emphasized the various ways in which American society ignores, denies, misinterprets, and even promotes suffering. America, however, also spends more money than any other nation on the care of the sick. This country has done as much as, if not more than, any other nation to include people with disabilities in our public and private systems. The Americans with Disabilities Act of 1990, for example, signified our commitment to integrating those with disabilities into more facets of American life. We have also brought about some of the world's most sweeping changes in disease prevention; witness smoking bans and speed limits.

Thus, America as a whole is not completely insensitive to suffering, but it could definitely enhance its sensibilities, personally and institutionally, to suffering as a universal fact of life. Implementing prescriptions to heighten our sensitivity would be difficult and complicated. Recognizing that the insight, analysis, dialogue, and understanding necessary to undertake such a task is far beyond the scope of this discussion, I nonetheless attempt some suggestions, with the hope that they will at least offer a starting point.

Acknowledge Suffering

First, we need more discussion about suffering and its meaning in our individual lives and in our culture. A nation of optimists, expansionists, and youth and beauty idolaters, ours is a society naturally hard-pressed to think of life as a dance with illness and death. Yet, talking and thinking about suffering are important steps toward removing the taboos and restoring suffering to the human condition, as well as to the community at large. The American myth that it takes a strong will to avoid suffering needs to be reshaped to fit reality, namely, that suffering is the inescapable stuff of life that we can work to minimize and seek to prevent wherever possible but cannot completely eliminate from anyone's life. Suffering is shared by all of us and, as such, could serve as an inclusive, uniting force rather than as a divisive, exclusive, or alienating influence. Thus, instead of increasing the suffering of friends by ignoring their plight, we need to seek out such friends and help end their isolation. Acknowledging suffering does not make it go away, but it lessens a person's painful separation from the world that suffering often imposes.

Second, this nation needs to find a way to integrate its traditional values with a less superficial understanding of individuality and the concomitant hope for a long, painless, blemish-free existence unencumbered by the responsibilities of social ties. Self-sufficiency has been overemphasized; we cannot continue to neglect our need for community, especially when dealing with illness and suffering.

Health care professionals are in a good position to apply the above approaches where they are most likely to have significant impact. Indeed, their responsibility to treat illness implies the need for their attention to suffering, or the "hidden dimension of illness." The social, psychological, and even religious spheres out of which suffering is borne define what it means to be ill just as do genetic aberrations and physiological malfunctions. Caregivers who work to heal by uncovering the physical origins of disease also should discover and address the fuller panoply of concerns associated with illness.

Join Behavioral and Physical Sciences

For health care professionals, a major step in addressing suffering may be to incorporate in their ethic the side of human nature that comprises the emotional, aesthetic, and spiritual dimensions of personality. The "Seldin solution" must be replaced with a broader view of science and healing and a more flexible border between the science and art of medicine. Science seems to be moving in this direction; more and more biomedical scientists are beginning to agree that expanding the paradigm beyond the Newtonian concepts should not compromise their ability to continue to mine reductionist theory for as-yet undiscovered treasure. This new movement in biomedicine—partly because of its insistence that the scientist-observer cannot only be considered an external, objective observer, but a part of the experiment—may help bring behavioral science into full intellectual partnership with the academic health community. Movement in this direction will also expand awareness of the importance of dealing constructively and openly with suffering within the overall health care enterprise.

Health care professionals should also endeavor to educate themselves formally about suffering. The volume of literature in this area is small but, fortunately, growing as the impact of the social context of illness is increasingly appreciated. AIDS has opened up a national discussion about suffering and has helped to demystify the subject; AIDS literature, particularly that written by people with

AIDS themselves, has much to teach about suffering. Those who have studied suffering have observed common phenomena of which every health care professional should be aware, namely, that the degree of suffering a person experiences has little to do with the intensity of the physical pain, and that suffering is often masked by apathy, which can reflect hopelessness rather than a lack of motivation to get better. In this regard, the work of Eric Cassell, Arthur Kleinman, nursing dean Patricia Starck, and others who have sought to understand suffering is well worth contemplating.

Physician, Know Thyself

Caregivers should also take stock of their own biases, interests, and emotions and consider how these may color their perceptions of patients and their suffering. You might ask yourself, "What constructs comprise my beliefs about suffering? That it is divine punishment for transgression? That it signifies personal weakness?" Negative childhood experiences with an alcoholic parent, for example, may have rendered you unsympathetic to the suffering of addiction. Perhaps your upbringing has instilled in you a simplistic view of the suffering of members of other racial and ethnic groups. Maybe you have a particularly high tolerance for pain or for solitude, and, therefore, risk discounting the factors that elicit suffering in others.

I know that my excessive and immature fear of dependency on others once interfered with my ability to care adequately for quadriplegic patients. When I worked through my feelings, I improved as a caregiver. Understanding the lenses through which we view the world can help us discern more clearly the nature of the images we see through those lenses.

Health care professionals also must monitor their own physical and emotional energy levels and consider how these levels may be affecting their interactions with patients and their capacity to recognize and respond compassionately to suffering. The chaotic urban emergency room provides a salient example of a setting in which desensitization and burnout may keep professionals from recognizing suffering. Frustration and exhaustion can easily overwhelm compassion; the importance of taking time for self-renewal cannot be overemphasized.

Humanize the Environment

Institutional environments such as emergency rooms and intensive care units can also complicate the recognition and management of suffering. The whirring and beeping machines of medicine not only focus the practitioner's attention on the physiologic processes of illness, but also can intimidate patients and their families as they try to contemplate illness, loss, and perhaps even death. Caregivers should seek to minimize the negative effects of such environments, to make time and space for the low-technology, less tangible aspects of care.

When a practitioner finds it difficult or impossible to ease a patient's emotional suffering, that practitioner should be aware of other support systems in the community—other health professionals, counselors, clergy, support groups, community activities—with which the patient may be connected. Just as the caregiver follows up on biomedical interventions, he or she should also follow up on these other interventions.

Initiate and Maintain Communication

Perhaps the most overlooked, but most powerful, tool for handling suffering is communication. It sounds so simple—asking patients, in one way or the other, if they are suffering. But many caregivers apparently fail to do so. It may be that they feel their primary responsibility is to address physical conditions, a complex and exhausting task. It is more likely, however, that they shy away from addressing this issue because it is difficult and unpleasant.

The power of communication to alleviate suffering is illustrated most clearly by the practitioner clarifying a patient's erroneous belief (for example, "I'll never be able to walk again with this artificial hip") and helping this patient to understand the exact nature of the condition, treatment, and prognosis (for example, "You will be back on your feet in a matter of weeks").

Perhaps more often, an understanding and alleviation of suffering require communication at a different level—communication about the significance or meaning of an illness in an individual's life. Is the patient who has had hip replacement an active person who gets great pleasure from physical activity and independence? Could weeks of inactivity and dependence on caregivers precipitate a clinical depression? Does it matter that the patient with a particular disorder is of one particular ethnic group or another? Does it matter to the therapist if the patient is a man or a woman?

Arthur Kleinman encourages health care professionals to act as ethnographers. Writes Kleinman:

> To the extent possible, the doctor tries to understand (and even imaginatively perceive and feel) the illness as the patient understands, perceives, and feels it. . . . By putting himself in the position of the family members and important people in the wider social circle, the physician can empathetically witness the illness as they do. This

experiential phenomenology is the entree into the world of the sick person. . . . The interpretation . . . deepens the clinician's understanding of the experience of suffering.

Perhaps the final note about alleviating suffering should be one raised by Howard Brody, who points out that suffering is maximized when patients feel that they are not respected by caregivers and others around them. At the very least, physicians and other caregivers must show their patients that they value and respect them as individuals.

Chapter Three

The Doctor as Patient—Why Mercy?

Marcus Borg is a modern New Testament scholar whose books attempt to explore Jesus' life and words in the context of Jesus' own times. This leading biblical scholar says that Jesus called on people to treat others with compassion. Borg asserts that the word that Jesus used for compassion—wombness, as translated from the Hebrew—refers to the love of the womb and, with it, a mother's encircling concern for and support of her child; over the centuries, the term wombness has become the word mercy.

This rich meaning for the word mercy first clicked for me when I was rereading a passage from Thomas Merton's writings, in which he crystallizes the meaning of his life's spiritual journey in the words that all novitiates say upon entering the Trappist order of monks. Merton himself had uttered these words when he began his long, complex, and now very public journey into the life of the spirit. In answer to the ritual question, "What do you ask?" Merton gave the ritual answer, "I ask for the mercy of God and of the Order."

Thanks to Borg, I understand Merton's message in a new light: Merton is seeking compassion from his brothers and from God. I also have made a new connection regarding patients and the role that the health care system plays in our society. When gravely ill, suddenly disabled, or near death, even the most autonomous, independent, and strong among us seek the mercy of our society through our individual caregivers and the organized health care delivery system. Anyone may need such compassion one day.

Yet, compassion requires time. With health care time inordinately rationed today in the interest of economy, Americans could organize themselves right out of compassion.

For thousands of years, cultures have assigned high status and special designations to their healers and usually have leaned heavily on the intervention of the healer's compassionate efforts

to help their patients. It would be a tragedy, just when we have so many effective scientific ther-
apies at hand, for scientists to negotiate away the element of compassion, leaving this crucial
dimension of healing to nonscientific healers. In other words, we scientifically trained healers
must develop and sustain health care delivery venues that allow us to show mercy when people
most need it—and that is, when they are suffering!

Facing a Life-Threatening Illness

Two years ago, my life unexpectedly entered a totally new phase. I went for a CT scan of my mediastinum (the space behind the heart). A right middle-lobe bacterial pneumonia I had experienced some months earlier was resolving more slowly than normal. To everyone's horror, the scan revealed a large mass behind my heart that seemed to encircle the right main-stem bronchus leading to the right lung. The list of possibilities included tumors that would scare anyone and called for prompt diagnosis, which meant a thoracotomy and biopsy. The eventual diagnosis, malignant lymphoma, required six rounds of identical therapeutic interventions with three major metabolic poisons and a short course of prednisone. Five months of treatment was followed by diagnostic tests to ascertain whether I would fall among the three-quarters of patients who have a good outcome or among the significant minority who face a more difficult future.

Thus, at age sixty-one, and for the first time since age seven, I was confronting a serious illness that brought me into heavy contact with the hospital and health care system as a patient rather than as a caregiver or administrator. This time I faced a more-than-abstract possibility of fatal disease and certain involvement with a systematic biologic poisoning that would, even if all worked well and without complications, cause chronic illness for the duration of therapy and the ensuing recovery period.

Today, as I write these words some two years after diagnosis, it appears that I have fallen into the group of patients who have experienced a remission and possibly a cure (the latter, of course, to be determined by time).

A Child's View of His Illness

My only prior experience with life-threatening illness had been when I was seven and stricken with an acute streptococcal epiglottitis that required an emergency tracheostomy. It was followed by an almost fatal double pneumonia. It is said that I was saved only because of the availability of sulfanilamide (one of the first wonder drugs and the chemotherapeutic agent that preceded penicillin in the late

1930s). Meanwhile, I truly believed that I would die, because I had heard many people say so for several days, and I had had the last rites of the Catholic Church, a sacrament I well understood, having just experienced my first communion.

Frankly, however, the entire procedure all seemed relatively painless to this young child and, in fact, bore many pluses: I got enormous attention from my family and was catapulted from being the youngest and last in the family constellation into the center of the emotional stage.

Three vivid images of the experience remain. The first is when my father was placed on a pallet about twelve inches higher than one I lay on, while we were connected vein to vein so that blood could flow from him to me (presumably because I needed some). It seemed clear to me even at that time that he was directly involved with saving my life. Second is the vision of Dr. Shapiro, the kind pediatric specialist who saw me through the pneumonia and sat head in hand on many evenings observing me for long periods at a time, almost as though he hoped his mere presence would help. (I think it did.) Third was the sense that I have had ever since then, but especially during the twenty years that followed, that I had escaped death and that I somehow owed something to others. For me, each subsequent birthday and life experience that I celebrate are gifts that would not have been mine to enjoy if all the right people and techniques had not been in the right place at the right time.

Three Physicians View Their Illnesses

Now, more than five decades later, having no real complaint should my life expectancy become somewhat truncated, I might reasonably expect an illness to teach me different lessons and to challenge me in different ways than in my youth. Struggling to make sense of the new experience and almost by serendipity, I stumbled on two records written by physicians, each of whom had also been stricken suddenly with a potentially fatal disease while asymptomatic and happily working away. The first is a brief account by John C. Vander Woude, a young cardiothoracic surgery resident, who was discovered, on routine examination, to have a malignant lymphoma. Because he was about thirty years old and close to the height of his profession, his disease posed a completely different threat to him and his family than the one that I faced. But his experience with the sudden transition from a high-powered operative, controlling the levers of the hospital, to a passive recipient of orders (just as I had encountered) enhanced his understanding (as it did mine) of what the patient goes through at the hands of a health care team and within the sometimes grinding gears of the hospital and overall health care system. For example, as a patient needing his blood drawn at the chemistry lab, he had to wait in line as a supplicant in a setting he used to dominate as a house physician.

Perhaps the most striking description of what a sensitive physician-turned-patient can learn and has to teach the rest of us is in a book by Fitzhugh Mullan. He suddenly discovered via a routine chest x-ray study that he had, much as I had, some unknown, asymptomatic tumor. In Mullan's case, however, the problem was much more severe than mine, the diagnostic process far more complicated and life-threatening, the course in the hospital and treatment to eventual recovery much more prolonged, and the ordeal far more anxiety-producing and trying for his family and his professional life. His story and its lessons are, therefore, that much richer and merit careful review by every caregiver and caregiver-to-be. One vignette from Mullan's story leads nicely into one of the major points that I wish to make from my own experience.

After an extraordinarily grueling, heart-rending struggle with cancer treatment and rehabilitation, Mullan was ready for discharge from the hospital's protective environment to what now seemed to him to be a threatening and strange outside world. He felt, perhaps for the first time, a strong desire to take his own life. Grappling with his feelings, he let the hospital staff know that he needed some help. Shortly, a staff psychiatrist arrived. After listening briefly to the distraught patient, the psychiatrist, in an apparently brilliant therapeutic insight, uttered only seven words, "Do you want me to hold you?" The words turned the entire situation around. The reader of Mullan's work leaves the scene with the vision of two men embracing; one giving of his strength to the other—embattled, scared, and suffering—the power to continue the struggle toward a return of well-being.

This striking story brought home what I had experienced in a less dramatic fashion (two times personally and professionally many times more), namely, the capacity of specialists who do not have frequent or continuing deep encounters with a patient to say or do the right thing at just the right time to hasten the march toward recovery. Over the years, I have encountered some of the reverse as well, but the lesson remains that both the generalist and the specialist have enormous opportunities to influence the course of a patient's treatment, in ways that flow sometimes from professional expertise and sometimes from human nature and personality.

Grateful for the latest breakthroughs. Without embarking on a long (and likely boring) self-analysis, it does seem useful now, as a recent patient, to summarize my impressions of the most important aspects of what I will discuss at length in the next chapters. First and foremost must be the extraordinary scientific and technologic advances now brought to bear on the patient's problems through the professional competence of the modern health care team. That may sound like campaign rhetoric by some apologist for modern American medicine, but it is a heartfelt expression of appreciation from a knowledgeable patient who was surprised at how easy and painless major diagnostic and therapeutic interventions could be. Advances in anesthesia enabled me to go to sleep so quickly and easily, so dimmed any recollection of postoperative pain, and so effectively controlled the anticipated postoperative symptoms that the thoracotomy and other surgical maneuvers are not unpleasant memories and were accomplished within a three- or four-day hospitalization. Surgical techniques (for example, the use of miniature cameras, reduced incisions, and newly developed professional skills) all served to minimize possible postoperative side effects and make the entire diagnostic phase minimally intrusive and destructive to my remaining strength and resolve to go forward aggressively with necessary chemotherapy.

The science and techniques involved with the chemotherapy itself were most impressive. New medicines successfully prevented the dreaded nausea and vomiting ordinarily associated with the protocol I entered, minimizing the discomfort and trauma of the repetitive poisoning. Needles used for infusions and the little technologies employed to achieve other routine goals were effective and are continually being improved. Products of our pharmaceutical industry were used to make my bowel habits as nearly normal as possible, to prevent gastrointestinal ulcers from developing, and to manage strange alterations in secretions resulting from the therapy. Although one may argue that we do not need all of those technical advances and that a patient could do without at least some of them, I can categorically state that I remain deeply appreciative for every last one.

Perhaps the most striking technological impact on my own case involved the CT scan of the mediastinum, which uncovered the lesion in the first place and is the best available venue for following the therapy's progress. Without the availability of the scan, my condition would likely have gone undetected for perhaps another year, while the lymphoma grew elsewhere and eventually produced symptoms that would allow for diagnosis by biopsy or other means. Who knows what the difference in outcome would have been if such a delay had occurred?

Who knows how high the total cost of my illness could have risen had such a delay been necessary? For my part, I say God bless the CT scan! And God bless the skills and technologies available to most patients in America today! I look forward to the day when everyone has access to these wonders.

Grateful for human support. The second, somewhat surprising finding was my realization of the enormous importance of human support from family, other loved ones, and friends. The cards, letters, telephone calls, thoughts, prayers, and positive sentiments all serve to underscore and encourage the commitment of the patient and family to do whatever is necessary to regain health. I have promised myself that I shall never again be reluctant to extend such support to others for fear of intruding upon a highly personal time. It is, in fact, quite the opposite. Native Americans have long appreciated the value of the tribe's support to the restoration of health; I now understand and appreciate that dimension far more intensely than ever before. In fact, I now realize that some physician colleagues grossly underestimate such support, focusing instead on the science and techniques they know they can apply to a given medical problem.

Retaining dignity. The third lesson that I learned (or relearned) through this illness involves patient empowerment, independence, dignity, and psychological space. If I understand psychiatrist Leston Havens correctly, his therapeutic objective is to create a relationship with his patient in which the two can figuratively coexist and meaningfully interact, but feel no need to invade or be invaded by the other. Implicit in this simple approach is an enormous respect for the dignity and selfhood of the other. Attention to this need is terribly important when patients are physically sick and threatened with dire and dreaded diseases. Being treated with respect by all of the important players during my illness not only helped me to handle the situation, but more important, enabled me to grow as a person. My wife, children, and other relatives all worked to help me act as I thought I should in managing the thousand little daily decisions. My caregivers also were assiduous in attempting to impart the best information and advice that they could, and then in encouraging me to make the decisions and to set the course.

Combining this sort of approach with overwhelming support of the group, skills of the professional, and high technology offers the best potential for effective interventions on behalf of the patient. There is no doubt in my mind that the lines begin to blur between the individuals who participate in this network of patient support and the health care institutions through which much of the work is carried out. The interface between individual caregivers and institutions can be highly constructive from the patient's point of view, or it can be quite the opposite. Both extremes occur, as do all of the permutations in between. Identifying and improving those less-than-optimal permutations define the agenda for the health care team and system in the ongoing attempt to provide technically competent and humane care.

The gift of mercy. Finally, I found myself unable to escape Thomas Merton's stylized response to the ritual question of the Trappist order, "What do you ask?" It was, "I ask for the mercy of God and of the Order." Secularizing the answer, it seems to me that, as a patient with a serious, life-threatening illness, I was asking society for mercy in extending to me through its health professionals, its institutions, my family, and loved ones the requisite help to deal with the difficult matters at hand, because I could not do it alone. Whether the helpers are office colleagues or hospital specialists, the sufferer needs their merciful concern and support. At the core must be a latticework of morally accountable, concerned health professionals whose time-honored commitment to the patient's welfare is so central to our system of care.

Therefore, in my opinion, the caregiver's professional essence is based on the sustenance of the principles inherent in the ages-old covenant between doctor (caregiver) and patient: The doctor is the patient's advocate, and the patient's welfare is paramount.

Clearly, in this postmodern world, the concept of the solo physician must be extended to include other health-team members. Clearly, too, this foundation is not consistent with a health care system that creates financial incentives for caregivers to serve a corporation's bottom line or their own interests by restricting access to care. In such settings, health professionals are no longer patients' advocates, but advocates of their employers or themselves.

My own illness has underscored my personal commitment to work toward a health care reform that preserves the special therapeutic bond between the professional caregiver and the sufferer, a bond that is central to the seeking and showing of mercy, one to another! I cannot escape the notion that the extent to which we succeed in maintaining the humanity of our health care system should be an important measure of the quality of our twenty-first century civilization. For me, then, the name of the health care game is, indeed, mercy.

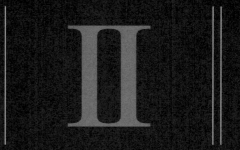

II

The Bedrock of Healing

Chapter Four

Language, the Other Arts, and Scientific Healing

Having introduced the distinction between disease and illness, I have also introduced the idea that pharmaceuticals and scalpels can address diseases. But to heal the illness and begin to reduce the suffering, something else is required. I believe that "something else" is the physician's communicating to the patient—by word, body movement, or other means of commitment—that he or she cares. This kind of communication can be rendered best by a caregiver who can decipher both the verbal and nonverbal messages that the patient conveys, and who knows how to respond to them appropriately.

It may be that some individuals are naturally more sensitive to the nuances of expression from others, and there seems to be a widespread belief that sensitivity cannot be taught. I don't believe that such biopsychosocial skills cannot be taught; nevertheless, there seems little doubt that faculty living predominantly in the biomolecular reductionist mode are often ill-prepared to either teach or exemplify such skills. Nursing curricula often address issues of interpersonal competency at practical and pragmatic levels. Physicians and dentists many times are so focused on the answers to particular questions, which lead them to decisions about the use of particular interventions, that they forget about the usefulness of the open-ended question and the value of giving patients a minute or so to express themselves. This latter approach not only uncovers crucial diagnostic information but is in itself therapeutic for the patient and may engender some peacefulness by uncovering and addressing such issues as anxiety, depression, and self-destructiveness.

Medicine: The Silent Art

Of the many forms of communication available to us, language is central to the development of the human species.* Physician Lewis Thomas identifies language as the most advanced and distinctive characteristic of our species. Cleanth Brooks, professor emeritus of rhetoric at Yale University, and I.A. Richards, a rhetorician at Harvard University, believe that language, as the medium for transmitting human value systems from generation to generation, is crucial to the development of a civilized culture. Where does medicine stand in relation to this primacy of language in the human condition?

Centuries ago, Hippocrates and his followers revolutionized Western medicine with their insistence upon observation, accurate description, interpretation of physical events, and intelligent intervention or nonintervention based upon their understanding of the patient's status. In so doing, they rejected language as an instrument for healing. An important part of that revolution is embodied in the phrase from the Hippocratic corpus that refers to medicine as the "silent art."

According to Pedro Lain Entralgo, professor emeritus of medicine at the University of Madrid, Hippocrates was reacting to shamanism, ritual chanting, and the practice of ancient healers to call upon the gods to resolve whatever was wrong with the patient. Hippocrates called for a retreat from use of the word in attempts to heal. He wanted his followers to observe, learn, and interpret before intervening in a manner based on their rational understanding of historical data and physical facts. The Hippocratic tradition then developed over many centuries as a stream of human activity separated from the use of the word in therapy. Doctors became doers, people of action, seeking to find new and better methods of intervening in the disease process. Talking, as a curative venue, had no place in Hippocratic medicine, and the dichotomy had to await Sigmund Freud for the start of some rapprochement between technique and word.

Paradoxically, in our retrospective and perhaps romanticized view of old-time country doctors, what physicians did have to offer to ameliorate suffering until the 1940s were mostly words. They personally stood by their

---

*This discussion is based on a speech made by the author at the University of Illinois Centennial Celebration: "Emerging unities of the twenty-first century: Service as sacrament, emotional neutrality, and the power of the therapeutic word." Chicago, June 4, 1992.

patients, guiding them through their illnesses and advising their families on patient care.

The Power of Words

Few would challenge the idea that modern medical technology has drastically improved our lives, even though it seems at times to be overly mechanical, impersonal, expensive, and frightening. One might even contend that the "silent art" should remain evermore silent, because it is simply not cost-effective for such expensively educated medical technocrats—today's doctors—to engage in the human support function.

Changed Biochemistry

An alternative argument can be made, however, based in part on the growing body of scientific evidence connecting the effect of a highly charged "word" on internal biochemistry. What we have begun to learn (or re-learn) about the link between the language arts and the soma suggests that physicians might well be overlooking a powerful therapeutic tool in words.

Among the modern advances in neurochemistry are many findings relating the emotional state of a person to the production of certain chemicals or the secretion of certain hormones. For example, the endorphins of the brain are endogenous, morphine-like substances whose production or secretion may be influenced by a variety of external influences. A large body of research also has been conducted on the debilitating effects of depression, stress, and negative emotions on the function of the immune system. It thus becomes easy to envision how doctors could use words as therapy if they only knew how to affect the patient's emotional state in an appropriate manner. I am certain that every accomplished physician has several examples from his or her own experience.

In *Anatomy of an Illness*, a book about his own serious illness that gave the author the opportunity to experiment firsthand with his ideas about emotions and health, writer and editor Norman Cousins provides one of the purest illustrations. He quotes Bernie Lown, a Boston cardiologist, on his treatment of a patient with an acute myocardial infarction. According to Lown, the most important therapeutic beginning can be the meeting in the emergency room between a recently stricken heart patient and an attending physician who soothes the patient by informing him or her that everything is under control: "You will be all right." Dr. Lown seldom has to administer the traditional shot of morphine to these patients, and they have taken an important initial step toward recovery. In this instance, it is clear that using the physician's words to create a trust relationship has been employed as therapy.

In a recent study, pediatrician and behavioral psychologist John Kennell and colleagues found a similar dynamic at work in the case of women beginning labor while accompanied by a supportive female companion called a *doula*. *Doula* is a Greek term referring to a woman who guides and assists a new mother in labor, delivery, and early infant care tasks. The *doulas* in the study were women who had themselves experienced a normal vaginal delivery with a good outcome, were comfortable with patients and staff from different backgrounds, and had gone through a brief training period to become familiar with labor and delivery procedures. In a controlled trial, the researchers found that the continuous presence of a *doula* during labor and delivery significantly reduced the rate of cesarean section deliveries (from 18 percent to 8 percent), as well as the frequency of the use of epidural anesthesia (from 55.3 percent to 7.8 percent) and oxytocin to augment labor (from 43.6 percent to 17 percent). *Doula* support also reduced the duration of labor and the rates of prolonged infant hospitalization and maternal morbidity.

The mechanism by which *doula* support influences labor, delivery, and perinatal outcome is not fully understood. Several studies in animals and humans have pointed to a link between acute maternal anxiety and disturbances in the progress of labor. It seems likely that a *doula* decreases maternal anxiety by her interactions with the woman in labor. Her constant presence, physical touch, reassurance, explanations, and anticipatory guidance make the woman feel safer and calmer and, therefore, in need of less obstetric intervention.

Kennell and colleagues suggest that medical costs could be reduced if every laboring woman had a *doula* at her side. Consider the potential savings: reduced use of anesthesia and other medications, shortened hospital stays for mothers and infants, and, most significantly, reduced cesarean rates and operating-room costs. Most of these factors could also translate into enhanced well-being for new mothers and their babies.

Norman Cousins agrees that positive feelings produce positive chemical changes that have true therapeutic value. While he was attempting to recover from his cancer, he experimented in watching tapes of humorous television shows and movies. He describes the effect: "It worked! I made the joyous discovery that ten minutes of genuine belly laughter has an anesthetic effect and would give me at least two hours of pain-free sleep."

Cousins also notes the slant of "psychobiological" research, or "psychoneuroimmunology" as it has come to be called, toward the study of negative emotions and their effects on health:

> Increasingly, in the medical press, articles are being published about the high cost
> of negative emotions. Cancer, in particular, has been connected to intensive states of
> grief or anger or fear. It makes little sense to suppose that emotions exact only penal
> ties and confer no benefits. At any rate, long before my own serious illness, I became
> convinced that creativity, the will to live, hope, faith, and love have biochemical signif
> icance and contribute strongly to healing and to well-being. The positive emotions are
> life-giving experiences.

Physician–Patient Interactions

Cousins emphasizes the importance of positive physician-patient interaction. He
believes that one of the physician's primary responsibilities is to help patients fully
engage their own abilities to mobilize the forces of mind and body to fight disease. Positive physician-patient interaction need not take a great deal of time;
many studies note that patients perceive a one- or two-minute visit from their
doctor to be much longer if their doctor sits down at the bedside rather than
stand in the doorway during the visit.

Empathy

Cousins notes that empathy is an essential ingredient in a healing relationship.
To stop and sit at the bedside is not only to show that you care, but also to enable
you to share the patient's experience of separation from the hectic pace of activity (which we often perceive as giving meaning to our lives) and get closer to
what it means to be bedridden.

Leston Havens describes the power the many forms of empathy (such as
tones of voice, gestures, and facial expressions) have in knowing a person and
helping that person heal. Of them all, he says, words may be the most powerful.
He calls language "the engineering structure necessary to translate passion (or, a
deep sense of caring) into what is clinically effective."

It is worth noting at this point that silence on the part of the physician also
can be a productive diagnostic, and even therapeutic, tool. On the average, it is
said, doctors interrupt their patients after the latter speak for only seventeen seconds. Aaron Lazare, Dean of Medicine at the University of Massachusetts, tells
me he instructs his students to give the patient a full minute and then five sec-

onds more to speak without interruption. He then suggests a follow-up question like, "Is there anything else?"

Using empathy in healing also opens new doors to therapists by increasing their sensitivity to the feelings and needs of others. According to Havens, "To find another, you must enter that person's world. The empathic visitor then discovers what he has taken for granted in his own world: that it is a world of particular time and space."

Related to understanding how patients feel is understanding what patients think about their illness and how treatment should proceed. Cousins, along with growing numbers of health professionals, believes that sharing the decision-making role with the patient is another mechanism through which the word can exert a therapeutic effect. The word is valuable in its capacity to enhance a patient's understanding of his or her condition and to reinforce a patient's sense of self-determination; both can decrease fear and depression and their negative physiological correlates.

Cousins writes, "If I had to guess, I would say that the principal contribution made by my doctor to the taming, and possibly the conquest, of my illness was that he encouraged me to believe I was a respected partner with him in the total undertaking." Surgeon Bernie Siegel concurs: "Participation in the decision-making process, more than any other factor, determines the quality of the doctor-patient relationship. The exceptional patient wants to share responsibility for life and treatment, and doctors who encourage that attitude can help all their patients heal faster."

In an earlier chapter, I mentioned a schizophrenic patient whom I saw when I was a fourth-year medical student. She had earned a Ph.D. at a major university; now she babbled unintelligibly, almost as if she were challenging us to understand her rambling. Over the course of several meetings, I was able to piece together her story, one that she directed mostly at the walls and the ceiling rather than at me. She told a tale of an ancestral princess who mistakenly had been abandoned as an infant among a group of lesser beings. These clearly subordinate creatures, although frequently kind to her, nonetheless saw her as ugly and inferior. One day, the princess's true father appeared. This great king recognized his daughter and placed a magnificent crown on her head.

When she reached this part of the story, the patient suddenly looked me straight in the eye and asked, "Do you understand?" I replied, "Yes. You are that princess, your hair is the crown, the rest of us are the barbarians. But I want you to know that I respect you."

My response seemed to satisfy her need to be respected and listened to, because this moment was pivotal in our work. She improved from that point on, perhaps because she knew that I respected her and wanted to participate in her efforts to work through her shattered emotional state.

These kinds of observations, by myself and by others, support the view that the physician should help the patient attain the best state of mind to cure him- or herself or to aid the external interventions in the curative process. To accomplish this feat requires a great deal of knowledge, understanding, and analysis of what makes some patients get well and others not, and how the doctor can influence the process by behavior and speech. Doctors should divest themselves of that part of the Hippocratic heritage that devalues words as restorative tools; it is an ideology that makes it difficult for many doctors to become true healers.

Bringing About Understanding

Why have more medical practitioners not effectively employed the word in their practice? It is probably because they were never taught that words in themselves can be instruments of healing. Medical sciences teach us that x rays, hormones, chemotherapy, antidepressants, analgesics, and CAT scans are highly effective tools and that words are not. All too often, we are uncomfortable with words, embarrassed by or ineffectual with them, and we see them as valueless in the fight against a tangible physical ailment. It is a disquieting situation: as the profession becomes ever more effective in utilizing science and technology, the public is becoming increasingly disaffected by the health care received. Physicians are accused of being inhumane, mechanistically oriented, and materialistic. Although most doctors realize at some level that their words can have tremendous impact, most caregivers do not think of the use of words as a scientific mode of therapy.

As physician Lewis Thomas relates, the modern hospital environment often seems entirely incompatible with "the therapy of the word":

> Today, with the advance of medicine's various and complicated new technologies, the ward rounds now at the foot of the bed, the drawing of blood samples for automated assessment of every known (or suggested) biochemical abnormality, [and] the rolling of wheelchairs and litters down through the corridors to the X-ray department, there is less time for talking. The longest and most personal conversations held with hospital patients when they come to the hospital are discussions of finances and insurance, engaged in by personnel trained in accountancy, whose scientific instruments are the computers.

In their handbook *Talking and Listening to Patients: A Modern Approach*, medical educators Charles Fletcher and Paul Freeling point out that there is ample evidence that patients are frequently dissatisfied with what doctors tell them about their illnesses; perhaps more serious is the fact that many patients do not do what their doctors tell them to do. Various studies have shown that between 10 and 70 percent of patients (and an average of 50 percent) do not take their prescribed medications and reject their doctor's advice about changes in lifestyle.

The history of communication between doctors and patients is interesting. Many doctors used to think it was bad for patients to understand their illnesses and treatments. "Good" patients did what they were told without question. "Troublesome" patients questioned doctors in a way thought to undermine respect for, and confidence in, doctors. Although recent years have demonstrated a shift toward sharing medical information more liberally, many patients still find it difficult to get all the information they want to have about their illnesses. They are frequently not invited, as many would wish, to help decide on their treatment.

It is clear that there is still much work ahead. In a recent study of physician-patient communication, J. K. Burgoon and colleagues conclude that the manner in which the medical practitioner communicates with the patient may contribute more to patient satisfaction than the content of the communication itself. The authors interviewed 234 adults who had seen a primary care doctor within the previous six months. They found that greater patient satisfaction was associated with more expressions of receptivity, immediacy, composure, similarity, and formality, as well as less physician dominance. In such consultations, patients trusted their physician more, believed the physician was concerned about them, believed they were well-informed, felt safe to disclose information, felt liked and accepted, and were more satisfied with the physician's techniques. These factors also had a modest positive effect on patients' compliance.

An Indispensable Diagnostic Tool

Good communication between doctors and their patients not only makes patients happy (and sometimes healthy), but also gives the physician the information needed to treat the patient effectively. Physician Philip Tumulty describes the dynamics eloquently:

> A clinician spends a great amount of his working hours communicating with his patients. What the scalpel is to the surgeon, words are to the clinician. When he uses them effectively, his patients do well. If not, the results may well be disastrous. . . . The

wisdom of Thomas Aquinas, the logic of Newman, and the clinical genius of Osler will not be effective in making well a patient who does not understand why he is sick, or what he must do to get well.

Physician Dana Atchley echoes Tumulty's thoughts:

> Warmth and compassion break down the barriers of anxiety and fear that beset the patient coming as a stranger to the doctor, barriers that can seriously inhibit the thoroughness of a diagnostic appraisal. If a patient feels that his problems are provocative, not only of scientific interest, but also of a deep concern over his happiness, he will be more open in discussing his life and his deeper feelings, and also more cooperative in accepting unpleasant diagnostic and therapeutic procedures. A good emotional rapport between the doctor and his patient improves his efficiency as a healer and, indeed, makes the whole process more pleasant.

George Engel, professor emeritus of medicine and psychiatry at the University of Rochester, is renowned for his definition of a biopsychosocial paradigm for medicine. In contrast to the seventeenth century scientific paradigm (accepted by scientists like Newton, Descartes, and Curie) that portrays what is being studied as external to and independent of the scientist, Engel holds that what is being studied is inseparable from the scientist. At the heart of the biopsychosocial paradigm is the notion that what a scientist (or a physician) observes is not nature (or physiology) itself, but, rather, the interplay between nature and ourselves— that is, science describes nature as exposed to our way of questioning.

Engel has described the patient interview, in which the doctor is the scientist doing the studying, as the most powerful, encompassing, sensitive, and versatile instrument in all of medicine. He believes that in an encounter with a patient, the physician must operate in two modes concurrently—observational and relational. Each deals with different sorts of data. In the observational mode, the physician collects data that can be observed through the senses (or extensions of the senses, like stethoscopes and blood pressure cuffs). In the relational mode, the physician collects data from the uniquely human realm of the interview, symbols, thoughts, and feelings. Through the relational mode, the physician learns the nature and history of the patient's experiences and clarifies what they mean to the patient and what they mean in other—psychological or social—systems. This clarification of meaning, achieved in the relational mode, illuminates measurements taken in the observational mode; together, they provide a clear, complete picture of the patient's symptoms.

Others agree that physician-patient interchange is the most potent tool for understanding a patient's illness and finding a treatment that works. In teaching medical students how to talk and listen to patients, Fletcher and Freeling divide the physician-patient consultation into two parts: the interview and the discussion, much along the lines of Engel's observational and relational modes. They emphasize the discussion mode:

> [D]octors should not just tell patients about the diagnosis and proposals for management, but should first find out their views and discuss them in order to reach an agreed diagnosis and plan of action. Studies have shown that patients will be more likely to accept and carry out this plan if they have participated in its formulation.

Fletcher and Freeling concede that good consultations may on average take more time than inferior ones, but if this means that they are more effective, they will save time in the long run.

The Language of the Fine Arts

Just as words can go a long way toward helping physicians understand people and their healing processes, so too can other forms of expression. The arts, for example, provide powerful means for communicating thoughts and feelings. Like laughter or verbal reassurance, music and painting can make people feel good—inspired, relaxed, content. The arts can be a healing force.

For the physician, attempts to understand or relate to artistic works of all sorts help develop a sensitivity to patients that, in turn, enhances the ability to decipher both verbal and nonverbal messages that patients convey. After all, the arts are attempts at communication of emotions and perceptions, precisely the skills in which an increasing number of patients find many modern doctors most deficient.

Psychotherapists frequently use art in therapy with young children, for whom verbal expression can be difficult. To understand their feelings better and identify possible sources of subconscious emotional conflict that may frustrate the healing process, some clinicians ask cancer patients to draw themselves, their treatment, and their disease. These drawings may facilitate treatment of patients who are ambivalent about receiving a substance that they subconsciously feel is poisonous. Once the drawing unveils the patient's subconscious resistance, the patient may be able to consciously alter his or her attitude toward treatment.

Art also can be a source of positive feelings and, hence, a stimulant to our own internal restorative mechanisms. As those who work in the arts are aware, when we create something—a painting, a sculpture, a dance—we experience the basic pleasure of bringing something to life and sharing a part of ourselves with others. In this way art is a life force, reminding its creator that he or she has the power to make things happen and is connected to others in our world. Such feelings of vitality, self-affirmation, and connectedness are precisely the sorts of feelings lost by people isolated by illness and the prospect of death, feelings that a caregiver can help to restore.

Jamake Highwater, a writer and artist, once told me that he saw humans as isolated, individual beings, who, like stars in the sky, blink silent messages to one another. To him, artists were people who are particularly adept at reaching others and thereby conquering the isolation through their art. Harkening back to the isolation of suffering, connecting with an artist can be viewed as good for patients as well as for doctors who need practice in successful communication.

The therapeutic value of art is gaining increasing recognition. Programs to bring artists-in-residence to health care facilities have been created, and a field called "health care arts administration," in which hospitals become patrons of art for its therapeutic value for patients, has taken shape. Architects of newer hospitals have designed them to be brighter, more airy, and painted in pleasing pastels; their hospitals feel more like places for healing than places for isolating the sick or dying. Research has confirmed that patients are measurably better off if their room has a window offering a natural view. As pathologist and biomedical scientist Guido Majno points out, it is difficult to rise above the daily routine when the eye cannot catch a glimpse of the sky.

The Language of Music

The expressive and healing properties of music are perhaps the most widely recognized among all the arts. Music therapy is an established health profession; its beginnings, according to music therapist John Beaulieu, can be traced back to the observations of a group of professional musicians who worked with returning World War II veterans. The musicians volunteered in hospitals with the intention of helping the veterans pass time pleasurably. To their surprise, the musicians began to notice that the patients who were regularly exposed to music showed a marked increase in morale and improved socialization skills. As their suppressed emotions found a safe form of expression through music, their depression lifted faster.

Founded during the 1950s and 1960s, the National Association for Music Therapy and the American Association for Music Therapy were two early professional associations dedicated to understanding the healing qualities of music and sound. Merged as the American Music Therapy Assocation in 1998, it certifies music therapists graduating from the more than seventy university training programs in music therapy; it also supports research and work to increase public awareness of the benefits of music therapy. Today music therapists work in hospitals with such populations as the mentally retarded, physically handicapped, and learning disabled, as well as with people suffering from cancer, heart problems, and psychiatric conditions.

Norman Cousins relates the experiences of two famous personalities with illness and music. One was cellist Pablo Casals, who experienced infirmities in his late eighties; when he turned to his instrument, he breathed easier, his fingers unlocked, and his back seemed to straighten naturally. Casals described his relief:

> I see Bach as a great romantic. His music stirs me, helps me to feel fully alive. When I wake up each morning I can hardly wait to play Bach. What a wonderful way to start the day. . . . I suppose that every musician feels that there is one piece that speaks to him alone, one which he feels seems to involve every molecule of his being. This was the way I felt about the B-flat Quartet ever since I played it for the first time.

Cousins also cited the experiences of the great missionary physician and theologian Albert Schweitzer:

> Johann Sebastian Bach made it possible for [Schweitzer] to free himself of the pressure and tensions of the hospital. . . . He was now restored to the world of creative and ordered splendor that he had always found in music. . . . He felt restored, regenerated, enhanced. When he stood up, there was no trace of a stoop. Music was his medicine.

In the 1980s, the University of Texas Health Sciences Center at Houston developed a program to bring the visual and performing arts to the center. I recall attending a brown-bag lunch in a medical school classroom at which the director of a local professional ballet troupe discussed preparation for the troupe's performance at the school the next day. I know nothing of ballet and am not a lover of the dance. Nevertheless, I learned more in that half hour about body language in particular, and nonverbal communication in general, than I had in twenty years of clinical and teaching practice.

The troupe director demonstrated the way in which her completion of a movement or gesture sent messages to the audience, and she explained how certain movements could elicit an audience response. Since then, I have become more adept at reading body language. I have also gained a new and apparently lasting awareness of how I use my body language with other individuals or with groups.

The Art of Healing

With regard to the development of a healing relationship or the use of words or other forms of communication as therapy, I feel certain of two points:

1. It is a humbling subject, which can engage any interested caregiver for a lifetime of learning and self-enhancement.
2. The ability to succeed at helping others help themselves ease their suffering or defeat their disease has everything to do with caregivers building trust and confidence in the patient, accepting the patient and the patient's predicament in a nonjudgmental way, and sticking with the patient until the situation is resolved. By what he or she does or says, the caregiver must demonstrate that she or he cares for the patient.

Thus, whatever interaction one can have and enjoy with language, art, music, and other forms of communication can only enhance, either directly or indirectly, one's capacity to be a consistently constructive, positive force in a patient's life. It all boils down to the so-called "art of medicine." Successfully communicating a sincere interest in improving the patient's condition helps the patient feel more comfortable from the start. The very act is "healing," for both the caregiver and the patient.

Chapter Five

Treating Disease and Curing Illness

Oliver Wendell Holmes, in the nineteenth century, said, in effect, that if all the medicines in the world were thrown into the sea, it would be bad for the fish and good for the people. A famous French physician of that same era is also said to have stated that it was important to use all new treatments as often as possible before they became ineffective. L.J. Henderson, the Harvard biochemist, is reputed to have stated, "Somewhere between 1910 and 1912 in this country, a random patient, with a random disease, consulting a doctor chosen at random, had for the first time in the history of mankind a better than fifty-fifty chance of profiting from the encounter."

The Placebo Lesson

Clearly, medicine has had its trials as well as its triumphs. Given the historical ineffectiveness—and, in some cases, danger—of medical treatments and procedures, what can account for the constant need, use, and perceived success of medicine throughout the centuries? The answer may be found in a review of placebos.

A. K. Shapiro defines a placebo as:

> Any therapeutic procedure (or that component of any procedure) which is given deliberately to have an effect, or unknowingly has an effect on a patient, symptom, syndrome, or disease, but which is objectively without specific activity for the condition being treated. The therapeutic procedure may be given with or without conscious knowledge

that the procedure is a placebo, may be an active (noninert) or nonactive (inert) procedure, and includes, therefore, all medical procedures, no matter how specific.

The placebo effect simply refers to the outcome, favorable or unfavorable, that a placebo produces in the person who takes it. Herbert Benson and David McCallie, both of whom are physicians and physiologists, point out that the placebo effect may be subjective or may have objective physiologic manifestations. These manifestations can include an increase in endorphins, which leads to a reduction in pain. Higher endorphin levels also lead to increases in the vitality and effectiveness of the immune system's T-cells and macrophages, which can directly ameliorate and sometimes cure disease. Benson and McCallie describe three factors around which the placebo effect tends to revolve: the beliefs and expectations of the patient, the beliefs and expectations of the physician, and the nature and quality of the physician-patient relationship. They argue forcefully for more research on the placebo effect based on its powerful potential to affect patients' health.

A recent survey of the literature by psychiatrist Judith Turner and behavioral researchers supports the placebo potential. They found that placebo response rates vary considerably and are often much higher than the frequently cited 30 to 40 percent. They also point out that placebos tend to have time-effect curves, with peak, cumulative, and carryover effects that resemble those of active medications. Interestingly, Turner and colleagues also note that individuals tend to be inconsistent in their placebo responses and that no "placebo-responder" personality has been identified. Their article is a useful resource on the critical role that the placebo effect plays in the evaluation of new medical treatments.

More and more, developments in modern neurochemistry, neuroendocrinology, and neuropsychoimmunology allow us to envision how, at a molecular level, emotions and beliefs can influence everything from white-cell function to cardiovascular events. It has become much easier to consider the art of medicine as an emerging science through which the adept practitioner encourages the patient's own internal pharmacy to dispense agents in therapeutic combinations and amounts at just the right time.

The Placebo Effect

The essential mechanism of the placebo effect resides in the intersection of belief with pathophysiologic and molecular biologic processes. Simply put, a physician gives a patient with a complaint an inactive pill. The patient takes the pill, believing that it will relieve his or her symptoms, and it does. Not limited to treatment in the form of pills, the placebo effect can occur after any treatment, even surgery, that the physician and the patient believe is effective.

A number of studies on placebos and the placebo effect illuminate this fascinating link between psychological and physiological processes.

The first set addresses the phenomenon of voodoo death or "bone-pointing." The most interesting is a long essay by Walter Cannon, published in 1942 in the anthropology literature. Cannon describes instances of deaths among primitive peoples that truly seemed to result from the spells, sorcery, and black magic dispensed by "medicine men." Cannon brings unquestionable scientific credentials as a physiologist obviously sincerely interested in his research, and it is difficult to come away from the essay without acknowledging the probability that these mysterious deaths (mysterious, at least, to Western observers) did indeed occur.

Cannon described the bone-pointing syndrome as rooted in the tribe members' belief that they will die if a certain bone is pointed at them. The syndrome, which involves a rapid decline in health and then death, is initiated when a person of authority points the bone at an individual, or when an individual becomes aware that a punishable transgression deserving the bone has occurred. Death is surprisingly rapid even in previously healthy individuals. No intervention of Western medicine was observed to alter the downhill course of the syndrome, and no disease could be identified to explain the symptoms.

Cannon told of the case of a perfectly healthy young Maori man who began to die when he became convinced that, two years previously, he had been tricked into eating a forbidden food that was purported to cause instant death. Following this realization, the young man traced a rapid path downward, neither eating nor speaking. His Western friends tried everything to reverse the course of events, but their efforts were to no avail. Finally, they found the young man's tribal medicine man and bribed him to tell their friend that the gods had revoked the prohibition on the food he had eaten and that the spell had been removed. Near death by all physiological measures, the young man immediately brightened, began to eat and talk, and soon completely recovered.

Self-effected deaths have been observed in this country as well. For example, many clinicians recognize as almost commonplace the death of the remaining spouse shortly after one member of a long-married pair passes away. Modern articles on this subject have been written by George Engel, who studied rapid death during times of psychological stress, and G. W. Milton, who studied self-willed death in patients with melanoma.

Another set of relevant studies by researcher Stewart Wolf and his colleagues focuses on the placebo effect in gastrointestinal physiology and pharmacology. In one study, Wolf used pressure-recording devices to study gastric contraction patterns in several human subjects at rest, during digestion, and in times of nausea and vomiting.

In subjects stricken with nausea and vomiting, he was able to show that the administration of ipecac, a medicine that induces vomiting, had different effects based on the information given to subjects. When subjects were openly given ipecac, they vomited as expected. When the subjects were told that they were receiving an agent that would relieve nausea and prevent vomiting, their symptoms abated even though they had received the ipecac. Wolf concluded:

> Placebo effects which modify the pharmacologic action of drugs or endow inert agents with potency are not imaginary, but may be associated with measurable changes at the end organs. These effects are at times more potent than the pharmacologic action customarily attributed to the agent. Thus the familiar difficulty of evaluating in patients new therapeutic agents stems not only from inadequately curbed enthusiasm of the investigator, but also from the actual physiologic effects of their "placebo" action.

In a subsequent study, Wolf and M.A. Pinsky studied the effect of an agent purported to reduce anxiety and tension in thirty-one patients with a variety of chronic disorders, all with a heavy overlay of symptoms related to anxiety and tension. Each patient was alternately given a placebo and the test agent in a manner blind to both patient and physician. The researchers found that regardless of whether the treatment was the test agent or the placebo, about 15 percent of the patients got better, 70 to 75 percent stayed the same, and 10 to 12 percent got worse after each treatment.

Many of the subjects had vague and nonserious symptoms. Three had major reactions. One had overwhelming weakness, palpitation, and nausea within fifteen minutes of medication, regardless of whether the treatment was the test agent or the placebo. A second patient developed a diffuse, itchy rash after ten days of medication; when the medication was stopped, the rash disappeared, and the patient refused to participate further, even though the rash had occurred as a result of a placebo administration. The third patient experienced several symptoms, including watery diarrhea, within ten minutes after taking the pills; this patient experienced the same symptoms on three separate occasions after taking the pills, which turned out to include the placebo. These findings point to the power of the mind to effect real, and sometimes dramatic, physical symptoms.

A set of studies focusing on the relationship between psychology and physiology is summarized in a 1989 research briefing published by the Institute of Medicine of the National Academy of Sciences. The report concludes that substantial scientific evidence exists that behavior influences the immune system, both directly and through the endocrine system. The report relates the finding, for example, that bereaved men exhibit a decrease in immune system competence immediately following the deaths of their wives.

Others have uncovered similar connections. Researchers Janice Kiecolt-Glaser and Ronald Glaser, in their study on psychological influences on immunity, reveal the relationship between stressful life events and changes in the strength of the immune system. Neuroscientist Candace Pert and her colleagues build a case for the existence of a communications network of chemical interactions mediated by neuropeptides and their receptors, which join the endocrine glands, the brain, and the immune system in what amounts to the "biochemical substrate of emotion."

The patient's faith in the doctor, not in the pill, seems to be the most powerful force operating in the placebo effect. Bernie Siegel describes the role of the faith healer in primitive medicine and the somewhat analogous role of the modern Western physician as a source of inspiration for self-healing:

> Nearly all so-called primitive medicines use the placebo factor via rituals that foster assurance in the healing force, whether it is defined as an external god or an internal energy. Faith healing relies on the patient's belief in a higher power and the healer's ability to act as a channel to it. Sometimes a mere artifact or saint's relic is conduit enough. For a believer a bottle labeled Lourdes Holy Water has healing properties even if there's only tap water in it. . . . This is why it's so important that a physician have . . . the ability to project confidence. A patient's hope and trust lead to a "letting go" that counteracts stress and is often the key to getting well.

AUTHOR'S NOTE: A patient's faith in the doctor can also produce negative effects. Critically ill patients, for example, often ask their doctors how much longer they can expect to live, and their doctors often consider the odds and come up with a number. In many cases, patients who trust their doctors die right on schedule, as if to validate their doctor's prediction, even when, given their actual physiological condition, they might have lived longer. In light of this phenomenon, many observers believe that physicians make a serious mistake when they yield to the temptation to give such time prognoses.

Debate About Placebo Use

Why then, when many studies on the placebo effect suggest that placebos lead to a 30 percent to 40 percent (some claim 50 or 60 percent) improvement rate in almost any symptom, has this important tool been ignored for so long?

Since the Second World War, what we may appropriately call the biomolecular revolution has swept forward with dramatic results, touching virtually all of our lives. The words "one gene, one enzyme, one protein, one disease, one precise cure" describe the concept of reductionist biomedicine at its best. This paradigm has produced increasingly effective tools, which have been so dramatic that all of us have focused on the tools and not on the healer or the healed. The Human Genome Project, which for the last decade has progressed ahead of schedule in its effort to map the entire human genome, with all the incredible potential it entails, is perhaps the ultimate expression of the reductionist theory.

Generations of doctors have been trained under the pervasive influence of the tremendous successes of the biomolecular revolution, which seems to extend the promise of perpetual improvement. In that context, physicians have come to regard placebos and the placebo effect in a cavalier manner, if not with outright disdain. Many mature physicians consider that a patient cured by placebo is somehow something less than a "real" patient and that a doctor whose work is done through the placebo is less than a "real" doctor.

It is true that Americans have a strong belief in high technology. We believe in our capacity to control or intervene artificially. Our faith in interventionist technology should be challenged by the abundant and increasing evidence that most acceptable and standard medical practice consists of interventions whose effectiveness has not been statistically proven. Recent exploration of the placebo effect in and of itself has probably had a positive impact on the health of patients by placing renewed emphasis on the quality of physician-patient interaction. Physician Howard Spiro describes this impact:

> [W]e physicians live in two worlds: the world of science, which provides us with our ideals and with the real advances against disease, and the world of people, persons with instincts, with pain, suffering, hope, and joy. We have a hard time separating out what we learn in science from what we need in practice to deal with people. The placebo reminds us to focus on the interface between those two worlds.

Spiro adds, "What the placebo effect does is to act as the symbol of a connection—tangible evidence that some person cares and will try to do something."

In a recent issue of the *Annals of Internal Medicine*, William Zinn reports on the transference phenomenon in the physician-patient relationship and its power to affect health:

> Transference is a process in which individuals displace patterns of behavior that orig-
> inate through interaction with significant figures in childhood onto other persons in their
> current lives. It is a powerful determinant of patient behavior in medical encounters.
> Transference can affect the kind of physician-patient relationship a patient seeks and his
> or her response to interventions prescribed by physicians. . . . Transference issues can also
> affect level of somatization and patient adherence to medical regimens.

Some have expressed concern about complications that placebo use may introduce into the caregiver-patient relationship. Author and lecturer in philosophy Sissela Bok argues categorically that giving a placebo to a patient constitutes an overt act of trickery and, however well intentioned, constitutes an unethical act. She refers largely to situations in which doctors give patients "sugar" pills or other inert substances, claiming that the substances are medication. If our understanding of the placebo effect is broadened, however, to take into account that it can occur with any therapeutic intervention involving either inert or active substances, then the physician giving medicine with an obvious hope that it will improve the patient's condition clearly seems acceptable.

As debate about the ethics of placebo use persists, other potential problems created by placebo treatment are clear. Spiro describes some of the practical hazards of placebo use by physicians; one of the most serious is that physicians may delude themselves into thinking that their patient has no significant disease because it was a placebo that successfully relieved the patient's pain. The physician may also mistakenly conclude that a placebo response means the original complaint was feigned. In either case, successful placebo treatment can engender false security or complacency in future instances of disease in a particular patient. In my own view, deliberate use of inert substances as placebos is a serious threat to the integrity of the clinician-patient relationship and should be avoided.

Learning More About the Mind-Body Relationship

In sum, we seem to have come full circle. Our modern science has generated spectacular new technologies, many of which are commonly accepted but largely unproven in terms of effectiveness, especially in comparison to the placebo effect or to other, perhaps less costly, interventions. Frequently, these technologies are practices in which physicians—and the public—place faith. Some future anthropologist may well conclude that our current American health care system is merely a high-tech, highly interventionist, specialty-oriented enterprise that is actually a giant, super-sophisticated, highly mechanized placebo. If so, we must sustain at least the 40 percent effectiveness of the placebo effect and not squander the public trust, thereby reducing this success rate. On the other hand, no reasonable person doubts the wonderful contributions of modern science to diagnosis, therapy, and prevention. Our evolving sciences show every sign that our laboratories will continue to issue truly effective therapies. Equally important is using our science to learn all that we can, as quickly as we can, about the mind-body relationship. If we can understand how an individual's beliefs can enable the patient, and not the doctor, to effect a cure, then we have hit on real healing that could provide us with the means to teach others how to heal themselves.

Chapter Six

Death and the Caregiver

There was a soft gurgle, followed by a gush of clear fluid that poured out of her mouth and onto her chest.

"She's dead," I thought. "My first death."

The intern standing next to me, in his second week at the Boston City Hospital, rushed off confusedly to try to do something about it. She was his patient. She was dead. The year was 1960 and I, a fourth-year medical student with no ultimate responsibility, actually accepted the fact of her death before the intern did. It was an awesome experience. I had finally witnessed that which all medicine is aimed against.

Like most of us, I wanted never to lose my respect and sense of awe for death. I vowed that at each subsequent deathbed I would recall, or try to recall, some of the feelings that had moved me this first time.

One week later, we students on that rotation rushed down the ward to the bedside of an apneic, cyanotic, cardiac patient, aged 65. An intern was thumping the patient's chest. I tried to figure out what I would do next were I the intern. The epinephrine was injected into the patient's heart. I was waiting and hoping for my first open thoracotomy. But the intern decided against the emergency procedure.

I was disappointed. The patient's heart had stopped; if he had held out a few minutes longer, there might have been a thoracotomy.

Another student ran to get an ophthalmoscope to try and see what was happening in the fundi at the hour of death. My interest picked up again. He returned and looked in. Then it was my turn. Zealously, I pulled back the dead lid, satisfied in my pursuit of knowledge, happy with *my intellectual curiosity. I focused the ophthalmoscope and then saw, realized, remembered what I was doing.*

It is a curious fact that future physicians spend countless hours learning about life and how to preserve it; learning about diseases and how they can kill people; and yet manage to avoid thinking about death as easily as the next person. Surely, we are young; we have not really entertained the thought of not being. Nevertheless, it seems appropriate that we (the students), in some sense should be experts about death, and that we not misinterpret that eleventh medical commandment: "Thou shalt not get emotionally involved with your patients."

Our society, rightly or wrongly, for better or for worse, predisposes us to the position that death is the ultimate evil and to be avoided at all costs.

I wrote the above words many years ago. The occasion of witnessing death for the first time creates vivid images; my recollections remain with me to this day. Interestingly, in the four decades since I wrote these words, the personal impact of a medical student's—indeed, any person's—first experience with death has probably not changed a great deal.

The tenet that doctors not get emotionally involved with their patients still persists, as does the belief that the point of medicine is to eradicate death. But the winds of change, or at least a gust here and there, have appeared.

Let us see if some of my words of 1960 reflect aspects of medicine today.

It is obviously crucial to teach medical students the intricacies of every method or technique that might possibly bring someone back from extremis. It is vital that no potential life-saving step be overlooked, but it does seem somewhat symptomatic that few words, if any, have ever been spoken to us about how to help a [person] die. It is our duty to see that [s/he] dies "in balance," but no one has ever suggested that we ought to make an attempt to care for [her/his] psyche during [her/his] last hours. We all believe that it is poor medicine not to "treat the whole patient," and furthermore we will expend a great deal of energy in enhancing physical comfort in small ways, which may have no influence on the final outcome of the sickness—and yet it is not always noticed that a dying man or woman very often seems to have less attention paid to them than to the patency of the multiplicity of tubes that are entering them from every direction, and which will enable us to study posthumously their last, hopefully balanced, chemistries.

It is not always noticed that more real effort is expended to get autopsy permission than to see to it that the patient does not die alone. It is almost as though, as doctors, we express our denial of death by focusing our attention upon the tubes, the chemistries, and the autopsy.

We tend to regard our treatment as having failed if the patient dies. "Successful treatment" is a term too often reserved only for those who live. One could submit another category, that of the successfully treated terminal event. One could suggest that the physician throw off [her/his] scientific mantle when at the deathbed, and become something else—and that something ought to be whatever the patient requires. It is apparent that, for a physician in modern America to do this, he must be capable of dealing sympathetically with agnostic, atheist, Protestant, Jew, Moslem, or Catholic, and with what he may consider personally to be unreasonable, superstition, or sheer lunacy.

It is hard for a student to talk about this ability in a physician because it seems that experience, both external and internal, as well as sincere effort are needed before one can succeed in becoming expert (if indeed one ever can) at helping the dying person through [her/his] death. Here, if anywhere, is the greatest stronghold of the practice of the art of medicine; here, as in every other area of medicine, is what one accomplishes proportional to what one offers; here, too, is what one offers proportional to what one knows.

The Wounded Healer

In some senses, the death of a patient is an insult or setback to the physician. In his book, *How We Die: Reflections on Life's Final Chapter*, physician Sherwin Nuland considers what factors may underlie this perception: "Doctors are people who succeed—that is how they survived the fierce competition to achieve their medical degree, their training, and their position. Like other talented people, they require constant reassurance of their abilities."

Feelings of failure when a patient dies, even when the death is largely inevitable, may be responsible for this "wounded healer" syndrome. Doctors as a group suffer from stress far more than most other members of society and are more likely to have problems with chemical dependencies. In his best-seller *Love, Medicine, and Miracles*, Bernie Siegel writes:

Throughout our training we learn not to empathize with the sick, supposedly to save us psychic strain. . . .The emotional distance hurts both parties, however. We withdraw just when patients need us most. Nurses know how hard it is to find a doctor when a patient is dying. All our education encourages us to think of ourselves as gods of repair, miracle workers. When we can't fix what's broken, we crawl off to lick our wounds, feeling like failures. The distance also encourages doctors to feel invulnerable: "It's always other people who are sick, not me." When I tell a roomful of medical students, "Almost everybody dies," they all laugh; but when I say the same line to a roomful of doctors, there's dead silence. We become the best deniers of all.

However, whether a patient is terminally ill or faces a serious risk of dying in surgery, it is beneficial for the patient and the health care team alike (physicians included) to recognize, accept, and even discuss the possibility of death.*

As an intern, I cared for a tough, elderly, white man from Montana who had a serious cardiac condition. Without treatment, he could expect his health to deteriorate gradually to where he would have to assume a sedentary lifestyle, far different than the one he was used to on his farm, and then face a premature death. Open-heart surgery, on the other hand, could significantly improve the quality of his life or, just as easily, end his life. The patient chose surgery, and briefly returned home to Montana to put his affairs in order.

On the morning of the surgery, I stopped by to wish him well. Tears filled his eyes as soon as he saw me enter the room; I could barely extend my good wishes before escaping into the hall where I, too, began to cry. This episode made me realize that I had become so emotionally involved with this patient that it would not be appropriate for me to be part of the surgical team. Striking a balance between human compassion and clinical detachment is a challenge for health care professionals as they strive to accept that death is the natural endpoint of life. It is not easy.

The idea that doctors should try everything to keep the patient alive, even if being alive entails suffering further agony as inevitable death makes its way, is pervasive. Our increasing control over the timing or occurrence of death has positive implications for patients able to return to lives of quality, but it can also bring about frightening, painful, and prolonged death. In many cases, our technology has outpaced our spiritual understanding of death and our compassion for dying patients.

In addition, the environment for malpractice in our litigious society may motivate doctors to pursue every method of sustaining life, even when that course of action may be harmful to patients and to themselves alike. Nuland describes the dilemma posed by the almost endless array of technological treatment options:

> Pursuing treatment against great odds may seem like a heroic act to some, but too commonly it is a form of unwilling disservice to patients; it blurs the borders of candor and reveals a fundamental schism between the best interests of patients and their families on the one hand and of physicians on the other.

---

* On the basis of all I believe I know about the nature of the healing relationship, however, it would be a serious error to make physicians the agents of death.

Physician Timothy Quill writes of this same dilemma:

> When the possibility for meaningful recovery becomes remote, then burdensome treatment begins to feel more like torture than a difficult means to a higher purpose. If the decision makers successfully shield themselves from the true burdens of treatment or from the reality that a patient is dying, then medical treatment can unintentionally prolong and dehumanize the dying process.

Just as aggressive treatment in the face of inevitable death may give patients and their families false hopes or "cheat" them out of a more peaceful parting, it can also be demoralizing to physicians.

Nuland defines the drive of many physicians to understand the precise details of a patient's pathophysiology, make a diagnosis, and design and carry out a specific cure—sometimes without regard to the well-being of the patient—as "The Riddle." He writes:

> The satisfaction of solving The Riddle is its own reward, and the fuel that drives the clinical engines of medicine's most highly trained specialists. It is every doctor's measure of his own abilities; it is the most important ingredient in his professional self image. . . . A physician's driving quest to solve The Riddle will sometimes be at odds with our best interests at the end of life.

It is interesting to note that societal and patient perceptions of doctors can also energize the quest to solve The Riddle. People tend to believe that doctors' reasons for recommending certain courses of action are wholly scientific. It is easy to overlook some of the other motivations, such as the need to preserve their own image as healers and conquerors of disease, that may be at play in doctors' medical decision making.

Let us continue with my words from more than thirty-five years ago:

> *It is clear that we ought to be familiar with the concept that death is a cruel and utter end to some people, while only a transition to something better or worse to others, and that we ought to be willing to act accordingly in our relationships with our patients. It is also obvious that any consideration of death does become philosophical and theological, and is, therefore, rather subjective. . . . But there must be something more we can know, objectively, collectively, to sharpen our sensibilities, deepen our insight, broaden our background, and thus enhance our understanding of any given patient in his last hours.*

Evolving Perceptions of Death

An interesting historical account of evolving perceptions of death appears in a book by ethicist Daniel Callahan. Callahan relates how death used to be a familiar, steady, and routine part of daily life. It frequently took place in the home, amidst family and friends who gathered to give meaning to the dying person's final moments and, as Callahan supposes, to show communal solidarity in the face of death. Prior to the rise of scientific medicine in the eighteenth century, medicine could do little to alter the course of critical illness, and death from illness was an openly accepted part of life.

With scientific medicine has come new medical tools and increased life expectancies. New beliefs about death also have begun to take shape; people no longer see death as a fixed, collective destiny, but as a personal tragedy, preventable or at least delayable. Where death was once a public event, it is now a private event, somehow ugly or shameful. People feel the need to sanitize the experience; families have begun to take their dying relatives to hospitals and nursing homes to die. Doctors often lie to dying patients to spare them the agonizing anticipation of death. In all of society, death has become a topic that is rarely discussed.

Although we have begun to explore the meaning of death in our modern society and to wonder whether we have perhaps made coping with death more difficult by shrouding the event in secrecy, we have yet to integrate death fully into our collective psyche despite its inevitability. Callahan writes:

> Death has not come out of the closet; only its foot is showing. . . . For all of its great triumphs, contemporary medicine does not know what to make of death. The end of life represents a troubling, and particularly recent, vacuum in its thinking. Death has no well-understood place in medical theory, even if it remains omnipresent in practice.

The Rescue Credo

The anxieties and ambivalence of the public and the medical profession over the handling of death feed one another, and technological advances continue to cloud the situation by proffering a myriad of technologies that can prolong and even substitute for many of the body's physiological workings. Callahan continues:

> There may even be a rising degree of anxiety about dying based on the growing difficulty in making a clear determination that a patient is dying, and that nothing more of life-extending benefit can be done. It is exacerbated by a widespread fear that modern medical death can strip a person of choice and dignity.

It is not merely the availability of new medical technologies that has complicated issues around death. Perhaps more important is the coupling of this availability with a belief that new technologies must be maximally employed, a belief that has been called the "rescue credo" of high-tech medicine. This credo is particularly influential when the patient's prognosis or wishes are unknown; in such cases, the credo dictates that physicians err on the side of aggressive medical treatment. As Timothy Quill explains, the rescue credo has its origins in emergency medical care, and he suggests that is probably where it should stay:

> There is a "presumption to treat" in medical care that protects physicians if they initiate emergency, potentially life-saving medical treatment in good faith on a patient in an emergency without the patient's knowledge or prior agreement. However, the presumption that all patients consent to medical treatment when their wishes are not known must be rethought in the case of the severely ill and the dying. Many times medical professionals feel forced to continue invasive medical treatments on patients whose wishes cannot be inferred with certainty, even when the effectiveness of such treatments is poor and the burdens are high.

Easing Out of Life

The medical mandate to prolong life clearly has its place, especially when aggressive medical treatment is likely to lead to a healthy, happy existence for the patient. In other cases, however, the value of the rescue credo must be critically evaluated. Patients unquestionably have the right to fight for life even when the odds are poor. But they should not be pressured to endure interventions that may prolong life while, at the same time, increasing physical or emotional suffering. Some would criticize those patients who do not elect to undergo every procedure that might buy another few days of life. Quill censures this as a harsh puritanical approach to fighting death that seems to pervade current medical thinking. "Going 'gentle into that good night' with one's dignity and sense of self intact," he argues, "is certainly as morally acceptable as raging 'against the dying of the light.'"

Despite the fact that the fear of lawsuits has added impetus to the rescue credo, physicians and other caregivers are increasingly appreciating the value of confronting death openly and of carefully evaluating the benefits and burdens of aggressive medical treatment. Many recognize psychiatrist Elisabeth Kübler-Ross as one of the first to break ground in this area with her 1969 book, *On Death and Dying*. Kübler-Ross espoused dealing with death and the dying patient sincerely and compassionately; her candid perspective is reflected in her own description of the book:

> It is not meant to be a text book on how to manage dying patients, nor is it intended as a complete study of the psychology of the dying. It is simply an account of a new and challenging opportunity to refocus on the patient as human being, to include her-him in dialogues, to learn from her-him the strengths and weaknesses of our hospital management of the patient. We have asked her-him to be our teacher so that we may learn more about the final stages of life with all its anxieties, fears, and hopes. I am simply telling the stories of my patients who shared their agonies, their expectations, and their frustrations with us. It is hoped that it will encourage others not to shy away from the "hopelessly" sick but to get closer to them, as they can help them much during their final hours. The few who can do this will also discover that it can be a mutually gratifying experience; they will learn much about the functioning of the human mind, the unique human aspects of our existence, and will emerge from the experience enriched and perhaps with fewer anxieties about their own finality.

The Hospice Movement and Comfort Care

Kübler-Ross's work was followed closely by the hospice movement in this country. Patterned after the efforts of Cicely Saunders, physician and founder of the hospice movement in Great Britain, the movement seeks to provide peaceful, caring environments without aggressive medical treatment for patients facing death. Hospice care takes place in special facilities (hospices) and, probably more often, in home care programs. A multidisciplinary team of professionals, including physicians, nurses, social workers, volunteers, and clergy deliver the care, often in concert with a patient's family members. Hospice programs have proliferated in the past twenty years, and in the mid-1980s they qualified for support under Medicare.

At the heart of the hospice movement is what has been called "palliative," or "comfort," care. Comfort care is a humane approach to the medical treatment of incurably ill patients that focuses more on quality of life, personal desires, and symptom alleviation than on prolonging life or treating disease. Although comfort care is most commonly associated with the hospice movement, it can be used in any clinical setting.

Unfortunately, comfort care is usually offered quite late, if it is offered at all—only after all possible effective treatments have been exhausted and the patient is near death. The care is usually presented apologetically (as if the physician has failed to help), rather than positively and as a legitimate and valuable approach to the last days of life. Comfort care is not frequently explored with patients whose quality of life is deteriorating and for whom acute medical treatments are increasingly arduous. Quill explains why: "For some physicians, the comfort care philosophy threatens deeply held traditional medical values. Many see their primary mission as fighting for life, and easing the passage to death has no place in that fight."

Many people who have studied death have observed that physicians sometimes even abandon dying patients for whom there are no more technological options. It seems likely that physicians remove themselves from the patient's bedside out of discomfort with death and their helplessness to stop it. Nuland relates this abandonment to The Riddle:

> As long as there is any possibility of solving The Riddle, [physicians] will keep at it, and sometimes it takes the intervention of a family or the patient himself to put an end to medical exercises in futility. When it becomes obvious, though, that there is no longer a Riddle on which to focus, many doctors lose the drive that sustained their enthusiasm.

To some extent, the problems of abandonment and oversight of comfort care options are probably rooted in the experience of medical education. On this point, Quill notes:

> In teaching hospitals, most patients are no longer seen by medical students or residents when the decision is made to treat them with comfort care. It is felt to be a waste of the trainee's valuable time when they are "not going to do anything." "Not doing anything" translates into not undertaking traditional, disease-oriented medical treatments; but by implication it devalues the many complex medical options still available to comfort the terminally ill. The clear message is given that caring for the dying has less importance than caring for those who will use medical technology to fight for life.

Nevertheless, it is certain that many mature clinicians know well the art of helping patients and their families negotiate the uncertain shoals of a certain death, without exposing everyone involved to expensive, uncomfortable, and ultimately futile interventions. A number of hospitals have recently endeavored to develop ethical and compassionate protocols for providing care to terminally ill patients.

For example, Texas's Hermann Hospital has developed a Supportive Care Protocol through its Program on Humanities and Technology in Health Care, led by physicians Stanley Reiser, Lawrence Tancredi, and Cheves Smythe. The protocol establishes clear guidelines for implementing decisions concerning supportive care for terminally ill patients. It specifically recognizes that "patients and their families (or other surrogate decision makers) may make decisions about health care that include changing, limiting, declining, or discontinuing a particular treatment, whether life-sustaining or otherwise."

The protocol* stresses that "the hospital's philosophy is to promote and protect patient dignity in the face of impending death by instituting medically appropriate care. Comfort will be maintained at all times through the provision of analgesics, hygienic care, and other appropriate medical and nursing care to all patients."

Protocols such as these reflect the medical establishment's increased willingness to deal with death and issues about dying patients. Medical schools have also made some progress in their approach to death. Many offer classes on death and dying, and a large body of literature has grown on the subject. The idea that the study of death could benefit from an emphasis on the meaning of death for individuals and societies, instead of on its physiological correlates, has received increasing support in the last three decades.

Finally, the American public is taking more interest in dealing openly with the subject of death and the unnecessary prolongation of life. Living wills, advance directives, and health care proxies, all of which give people greater power of self-determination, represent positive steps toward our society's acceptance of death. The recent exploration of death in the popular press, particularly Nuland's *How We Die: Reflections on Life's Final Chapter*, exemplifies the tentative steps we are taking back to a view of death as part of a natural progression of life.

Despite this progress, much remains to be done. As the Dax case (mentioned in a previous chapter) clearly shows, the refusal of the health care team to listen and to honor a dying or seriously injured person's express wishes remains common. The behavior of Dax's health care team is mirrored, to some extent, in the current debate over the propriety of physician-assisted suicide. We, as a society, have yet to decide that we will view death as a natural and inevitable occurrence, and that we will simply offer the dying the opportunity to depart this life in as humane and dignified a manner as possible.

Committing to the Patient

Physicians, nurses, and other health care professionals should try to understand

---

* Reprinted as appendix 4-1 in Starck and McGovern, *The Hidden Dimension of Illness.*

better the social and psychological aspects of death, and perhaps even some of the unconventional approaches to care that some find therapeutic. In this way, they can develop a more humane approach to caring for the dying. Good communication skills are essential to understanding a patient's wishes. Implicit in this two-way exchange must be a sensitivity to the value of patient desires in formulating treatment protocols whether or not those wishes are for aggressive intervention or comfort care. Encouraging patients to complete advance directives is one context in which physicians can initiate discussions about death and dying with their patients. Perhaps more important is the fact that advance directives relieve the ambiguity that can make death and dying in a medical setting so ominous.

Physicians must also explore their own beliefs about death. This self-reflection can help reduce personal anxiety about death. More important, it can enable the physician to neutralize more easily any overriding influence that the physician's personal values may have on treatment decisions that truly belong to the patient or the patient's family. Having contemplated their own beliefs about death, physicians are better equipped to handle situations in which a patient's wish to die may be explicit. In most circumstances, making certain that the doctor has the capacity to control pain and is not encouraged by external or internal pressures to overtreat is sufficient.

My own experience with dying patients has pointed to a seemingly simple, yet powerful strategy for dealing with death: fostering companionship. Often, just sitting by a patient's side is the best possible medicine for both physician and patient. I have seen how the presence of someone who cares, whether silently or with words, can significantly enhance a patient's well-being, no matter how grave the illness. So, too, can such companionship benefit the clinician.

Once, as a young student studying to become a physician, I asked an older physician about his most meaningful experiences in medicine. He replied that he found the most meaning in his role as a physician when he was with dying patients at the time they "turned around to face death." These patients shared with him a most honest and poignant moment, and his companionship, I imagine, enhanced their strength to accept and accommodate themselves to the coming end of their lives. Clinicians who decide that their presence is no longer necessary or useful for terminally ill patients, for whom no treatment options remain, sell both themselves and their patients short.

The experienced clinician realizes that all decisions, both diagnostic and therapeutic, are provisional and subject to revision as time passes and circumstances change. With this realization comes the understanding that the foundation of competent, continuing care is the clinician's commitment to stick with the patient, no matter what turn the course of illness takes. This is not an easy prescription, and the ability to fill it is a hallmark of professional and individual maturity.

III

The Broadening Scope of Health Care

Chapter Seven

Treating Individuals While
Tending to Populations

Our nation's health care system is being soundly criticized for costing too much and serving too few. Millions of people go without basic medical care because they cannot afford it. Miraculous operations (such as organ transplants) take place, but epidemics of preventable childhood diseases (such as measles) wipe out scores of unimmunized children. This situation illustrates a fundamental tension between American society's emphasis on individualism and our sense of responsibility for community welfare—derived from the American Constitution's mandate to "promote the general welfare." These words were written in the eighteenth century, however, and as time has passed, it has become far more complicated to take on this responsibility.

Many see the challenges facing today's health care system as a symbol of the rift between two professions that play major roles in maintaining health: medicine and public health. Claims that the health care "crisis" can be solved only through the union of medicine and public health are being figured into reform proposals, school curricula, and plans for allocating federal research dollars. There are calls for primary care doctors to practice in community health centers; for physicians and other health care professionals to counsel their patients about the link between behavior and disease; for medical interventions to be evaluated in terms of both patient outcomes and their impact on the burden of disease on the population; and for epidemiologic research to yield clues about preventable environmental risk factors and threats to health.

That public health and medicine should be partners in promoting and maintaining health seems eminently logical. So, insofar as we have not yet achieved the proper balance, where did we go wrong? The story begins with the birth of public health as a distinct endeavor.

Public Health's Beginnings

Throughout history, epidemics of such diseases as plague, cholera, and smallpox have evoked public efforts to protect the health of citizens through the isolation of ill persons and quarantine of travelers. Such efforts occurred even though epidemic disease was often believed to be a sign of poor moral and spiritual conditions.

> **THE KOCH POSTULATES**
>
> 1. The same pathogen must be present in every case of the disease.
> 2. The pathogen must be isolated from the diseased host and grown in pure culture.
> 3. The pathogen from the pure culture must cause the disease when administered to a healthy, susceptible laboratory animal.
> 4. The pathogen must be isolated from the inoculated animal and be the original organism.

At the turn of the nineteenth century, what was known as "the great sanitary awakening" identified filth as both a cause of disease and a vehicle of transmission. Momentous discoveries in the latter half of the century by such scientists as the German physician and bacteriologist Robert Koch, whose now famous "postulates" revealed the link between microorganisms and certain diseases, transformed the way in which epidemics were understood and combated. To this day, Koch's postulates provide a framework for the study of the etiology of any infectious disease.

The sanitary awakening, coupled with the birth and flourishing of medical microbiology, spurred an embrace of cleanliness and a dramatic shift in the way society thought about health: Illness came to be seen more as an indicator of poor social and environmental conditions and less as evidence of poor moral and spiritual conditions. These events also changed the way society viewed public responsibility for communal health. As historian Elizabeth Fee notes, "Poverty and disease could no longer be treated simply as individual failings." Public sewage drainage, waste disposal, and water purification systems were put into place, as were the voluntary hospitals that were a significant sign of community responsibility for citizen health.

As a result of nineteenth-century developments, pasteurization and immunization emerged as strategies for controlling and even preventing some diseases, such as tuberculosis and smallpox. The growing knowledge about sources of and strategies for controlling infectious diseases, and public acceptance of disease control as both feasible and obligatory, shaped the development of the field of public health.

Professional Turfs

Initially, medicine and public health were allies in efforts to maintain the health of communities. The two fields shared in their investment in epidemiology (the study of disease in populations), and practicing clinicians, in large part, made up the membership of professional epidemiologic societies. Ironically, the paths of medicine and public health began to diverge just as advances in bacteriology produced increasing evidence that the paths should merge. Not surprisingly, in the United States, tension over professional "turf" was at the heart of the matter.

Causes of Disease

The turning point in the history of the relationship between the public health establishment and the practicing clinical community came early in the twentieth century, when public health practitioners entered into direct competition with practicing physicians by offering immunizations. In *The Social Transformation of American Medicine*, medical sociologist Paul Starr relates a story about early twentieth-century tuberculosis control that illustrates a related point. He describes how requiring private doctors to give notification of tuberculosis to public health departments increased the tensions between medicine and public health:

> There was ordinarily no interference with patients under the care of private practitioners, and other consumptives were generally only visited by medical inspectors, who left circulars and gave advice about preventing the spread of infection. But fear of tuberculosis was widespread, and many people were anxious about any official report of its presence in their family; some life insurance policies were void if tuberculosis was the cause of death. Objecting that tuberculosis was not contagious, practitioners opposed compulsory reporting as an invasion of their relationships with patients and of patients' rights to confidentiality. The president of the New York County Medical Society told its membership in 1897 that by requiring notification and offering free treatment, the health department was "usurping the duties, rights, and privileges of the medical profession."

Public Health Evaluations of Clinicians

Another sort of tension that has separated clinicians and public health professionals is the growing tendency of the latter to function as assessors, evaluators, and critics of medical practice. An early example of this tension is the tragic story of Ignaz Semmelweis, the great nineteenth-century Hungarian obstetrician who discovered how to protect women from dying of puerperal sepsis after childbirth. Semmelweis observed different mortality rates between a clinic staffed by midwives and another staffed by doctors and medical students. He noticed that in the one staffed by doctors and students, clinicians were failing to wash their hands between pelvic examinations, and deduced that they were thus carrying infection from patient to patient and from autopsy to patient. Semmelweis further recognized the similarity at autopsy between death of puerperal sepsis and death of wound infection, and he emphasized the efficacy of handwashing with lime before attending deliveries. Finally, he demonstrated an extraordinary difference in maternal death rates in his own practice; his were much lower than those of his colleagues.

At that time, however, the medical community was unwilling to accept the link between handwashing and infection. For his outspoken advocacy against standard practice, Semmelweis was derided and effectively forced out of the profession. Broken in spirit, he died in an asylum, as young women continued to die by the thousands due to the inflexibility and closed-mindedness of well-intentioned, yet entrenched, practitioners.

The increasing role in medical care of what are now called the "clinical evaluative sciences" exemplifies the tension between clinicians and public health professionals today. The term refers to the application of epidemiology, sociology, anthropology, and statistics to the assessment of health care. As such, this research is often thought of as a public health–based enterprise. By its very nature, it is an activity outside the apparatus for the delivery of services. In many instances, what emerges from the clinical evaluative sciences is a tension between the active agent (the clinician) and the critic (the evaluative scientist or public health practitioner), with the latter telling the world about the inadequacies of the former. The tension is intensified when the clinician is someone who perceives him- or herself to be in the higher echelons of technical accomplishment within a specialty. Such a specialist may tend to criticize epidemiologic studies because the studies address the average level of competence—the collective success—and undervalue what the extraordinary surgeon or practitioner can achieve.

Politics

Political events also keep medicine and public health at odds. The relationship between medicine and public health soured further, for example, shortly after World War I, when public health workers tended to support national health insurance. Post–World War II federal initiatives in health care for the poor and elderly exacerbated already sensitive relations.

Organizational arrangements in education and service functions solidified the rift. The population-based sciences—epidemiology, demography, anthropology, sociology, economics, and health statistics—were relegated to the schools of public health, which were separated both geographically and ideologically from medical schools. State and regional public health departments were established separate from the personal health care system. Although relations between medicine and public health have improved in the past decade, suspicion, tension, and isolation persist in many sectors today.

Philosophical Differences

Paul Starr's account of tuberculosis-control efforts illustrates the friction between medicine and public health over professional turf. It also touches on something that has emerged as perhaps the most dominant force behind the separation of the two fields: the fundamentally different scientific paradigms under which they conceptualize and implement their activities.

Most physicians and medical school faculties operate under the Newtonian, reductionist, biomedical model, which emphasizes the understanding of disease and therapeutics at the molecular level. They tend to focus on individual patients, individual diseases, and the molecular interventions that will bring about particular effects. Public health practitioners, on the other hand, work with a variety of academic disciplines, the most important of which is epidemiology. Such professionals study populations, demographic trends, and overall morbidity and mortality statistics.

Thus, medicine focuses on disease and its treatment; public health focuses on prevention. Medicine strives to understand the diseases that cause poor health; public health seeks strategies to promote good health. Medicine aims to improve the health of individuals through specific therapeutic interventions; public health aims to improve the conditions of life for everyone in the community.

The struggle between the two fields boils down to a patient-centered approach versus a population-based approach. Seminal questions that involve both approaches are increasingly being raised by clinicians, third-party payers, and policymakers alike. One question may be, "Because individual patients are members of populations, couldn't their treatment be undertaken (to their benefit) in the context of what is known about the population to which they belong?" Most people would agree that the answer is yes. The growing number of medical conditions that we understand as having their origins in environmental, behavioral, and sociological factors make this strategy increasingly undeniable.

In the past fifty years, declining mortality rates from infectious diseases have been replaced by rising mortality rates from cancer, injuries, and chronic diseases of the cardiovascular system. The agent responsible for death or disability has shifted increasingly from the microorganism to the person. The most critical health risks facing populations are no longer contaminated water supplies and insects, but automobiles, drugs, industrial pollution, and diets laden with fat, calories, and salt. Awareness of these new morbidity factors makes obvious the need for teamwork between the fields of public health and medicine.

Kerr White, one of the most important and articulate advocates of the remarriage of medicine and public health, and medical professor Julia Connelly note that for most of the twentieth century, medical schools have had two predominant approaches: laboratory based and clinical. The laboratory-based approach is concerned with cellular and molecular disease processes; the clinical approach focuses on the care of one patient at a time. Although the value of what has been achieved in biomedical research laboratories has been tremendous— from early medical miracles such as antibiotics to more recent breakthroughs in organ transplantation—there has emerged a serious overemphasis on curative interventions rather than preventive practices. The overreaching curative gestalt of modern medicine has become associated with specialization, superspecialization, and an explosion of interventions and technologies to the exclusion, many argue, of other equally important considerations bearing on the patient's care and well-being. In the intense concentration on research and technology designed to unravel disease mechanisms in individuals, many people believe medicine has become overly disease oriented and has lost touch with the people suffering from disease.

In an essay on the role of physicians in health promotion, physician Robert Lawrence points out the tendency for some of the awe-inspiring technologies of modern medicine to overshadow many of the public health enterprise's intervention strategies, which are frequently less dramatic or glamorous. He writes:

In health promotion, we encounter issues of personal behavior, culture, values, and law. The triumphs of modern medicine are the results of experimentation and reductionism, of systematic attempts to remove all considerations of personal behavior, culture, and the like, to understand biologic systems.

Moreover, adds Lawrence, the more immediate feedback provided by successful treatment of symptomatic disease reinforces the physician's interest in pathology and therapeutics rather than in prevention or health promotion.

Health promotion and disease prevention present no "problem" for physicians; the emphasis is on health, on nonevents. Richard Pels and colleagues point out that health promotion involves "no dramatic surgical intervention, and the grateful patient is replaced by someone unlikely to credit, much less praise, the physician for improving the probability of a longer and better life." Moreover, the nature and scope of epidemiologic research can make its returns slow, although the returns can be particularly powerful.

Medical Education

Clues abound as to why the training of physicians has exacerbated the rift between medicine and public health. Most aspiring medical students load their premedical curriculum with the biological and chemical sciences, a pattern that continues into at least the first two years of medical school. Medical curricula lack sufficient formal exploration of the society in which students will diagnose and treat people when they graduate. From the student's point of view, a lack of knowledge in the so-called "hard" sciences (relating to curative medicine) can end up actually hurting patients, while a lack of knowledge in the social sciences would seem to have little immediate negative impact. Psychiatrist and medical educator Leon Eisenberg offers a possible explanation for the short shrift given to the social sciences:

There is widespread skepticism among physicians as to whether psychological and social factors are as "real" as biological ones. Classroom exercises will have convinced all of them of the power of biological reductionism. It is not only that so much more time is devoted to the natural as opposed to the "unnatural" sciences in medical education, but that the elegance of molecular biology is so much greater.

The infrastructure of medical education may also be a barrier to the study of communities. Much of medical education takes place at the bedside of sick individuals in tertiary care institutions, even though demographic and lifestyle shifts have greatly reduced society's need for tertiary care. Historically, outpatient service, the hospital's greatest link to the community, has been viewed as an "appendage" and a "charitable impulse," not as a site for medical education. Although positive steps have been taken to reshape admissions criteria, encourage the blossoming of community-based preceptorships, and create departments of community medicine, long-ingrained patterns are resistant to change.

Today, as always, physicians are trained to be problem solvers and to focus on the physical symptoms of the individual patient. Physicians are typically not trained to think in terms of prevention, health promotion, or social or psychological influences on health. In the words of one observer, physicians work in a "sickness industry"; this may explain, he adds, why they have been known to ignore things like child abuse, believing the issue to be none of their business. Although physicians frequently provide secondary or tertiary prevention services (for example, administering cholesterol-lowering drugs to prevent cardiovascular problems), the notion of primary prevention—that is, altering risk factors before they have even begun to influence human physiology in preclinical states—is something that most physicians still relegate to the domain of public health.

It is noteworthy that several studies report that physicians lack confidence in their ability to motivate behavioral changes in their patients, and they believe themselves poorly trained to practice preventive medicine. Lack of confidence typically correlates with little or no effort to counsel patients and with early cessation of counseling when working with less-motivated patients. Confidence levels tend to increase with the level of training. Surveys also document that physicians frequently do not adhere to preventive-practice recommendations because they perceive the recommendations as ambiguous or conflicting.

The literature can be confounding—comparable to, for instance, trying to discern whether butter or margarine clogs arteries faster. Part of the frustration may lie with the poor coordination between health services and the evaluative sciences, which are still in large part sequestered in the domain of public health. Evaluative statistical studies are often inconclusive and ambiguous, especially when it comes to working out the odds for a particular patient considering a particular intervention. Physicians also may find it difficult to assimilate new findings into their practices because of the rapid pace at which biomedical research moves forward.

Constraints of the practice setting can also hamper a physician's prevention and health promotion activities. Time pressures in busy primary care practices can interfere with delivering prevention and health promotion services. In addition, many practices do not have easy access to dietitians, smoking-cessation groups, alcoholism counselors, and other referral services that can help implement and provide educational support for health promotion interventions.

Joining Forces in Academia

Given the huge number of preventable deaths that occur each year due to cancer, cardiovascular disease, and tobacco and alcohol use, the great challenge to physicians and their health care teammates is to devote more attention to helping patients adopt healthy behavior. Increasing numbers of injuries, sexually transmitted diseases, and chronic diseases loudly signal the need for health care professionals to emphasize disease prevention and health promotion. Public health and medicine need each other. The separate contributions of these fields to improving the nation's health have been profound. Together, through the coordination of each field's unique strengths, public health and medicine could achieve even more.

Reshaping medical school curricula is an important starting point in healing the fracture between medicine and public health. Population-based concepts and skills must be taught to medical students; physicians need knowledge of statistics and epidemiologic concepts if they are to evaluate information effectively and efficiently. Equally important, knowledge of population-based approaches facilitates understanding of other vital elements that affect the natural history and management of illness. "Health of the Public," a medical education reform initiative of The Pew Charitable Trusts and the Rockefeller Foundation, outlines the need for instruction in diagnosis, treatment, and prevention to address not only the individual patient but also the community. It is within the community that the determinants of health and the factors influencing the severity of illness resulting from disease can be measured and modified. A number of forward-thinking medical schools have assimilated these considerations into their students' educational experience. More schools need to emulate this example.

Even if physicians working in managed care, health maintenance organizations, or other forms of organized delivery systems work largely on curing patients, they will need associates from nursing, public health, dentistry, and allied health to deliver preventive and health-promoting services. Thus, it is clear that the focus either on physicians or on public health professionals is too narrow to yield the best solutions. As we move to more organized and population-based systems of health care, we will be looking to the health care team to deliver the requisite services. Our educational and curricular reform should include all major health professions, not simply medicine.

Medical students and students of other health care professions need to be taught to integrate more fully the principles of community-based comprehensive care. Public health curricula, likewise, must make a serious attempt to engage the principles of biology, biomedicine, and reductionist biomolecular interventions. These interventions are especially critical; the ongoing mapping of the human genome opens the prospect that a drop of blood at birth can yield genetic information that will predict the disease and illness patterns to be experienced (and perhaps prevented) throughout an individual's life. The same genetics, now taught extensively in medical schools, will soon make clear to future physicians that they shall be armed more and more often with predictive risk information about currently healthy people so treatment can occur before sickness. Future physicians may be practicing preventive genetics! Thus, from a pedagogical point of view, more effective interprofessional teaching and learning should bring public health and medicine together. As students make choices between professional schools, they should include as a criterion the degree to which a school has been able to make this vital link.

It is clear that medicine must maintain the unique strengths of the medical approach. Nevertheless, the need for medical schools to be at the frontiers of innovation in technical and molecular medicine must not outweigh the need for the schools to shape their students and their services to meet the needs of the communities around them.

Similarly, schools of public health should maintain their unique strengths in epidemiology, health promotion, and disease prevention at the same time that they seek to understand better the basic principles and some of the more technical elements of biomedicine.

Balancing Curative and Preventive Care

Population-oriented public health professionals should also examine a phenomenon that I have labeled the "epidemiology of hope." I call it epidemiology because I believe it to be a population-based phenomenon; paradoxically, it also reaches the heart of the patient-centered medical model.

Each American, no matter how healthy, has the benefit of knowing that throughout every state in the nation are major medical centers where the latest technologies and the most proficient specialists are available should serious illness or trauma occur. This population-based hope allows us all to believe that if something dreadful befalls us, we, too, might have a chance at dramatic interventions and a typically American new beginning.

With some form of national health insurance coverage around the corner and health care dollars tight, a shift toward a more population-based approach to health care offers a certain appeal. In Oregon, for example, efforts have even been made to rank health interventions according to their public health impact—that is, according to how much "bang for the buck" they provide a population.

Prevention and health promotion activities have been emphasized in recent national health care reform plans because most of the time the costs of these activities are reasonable and their benefits are real. Part of the mandate to public health and other health professions is to continue to research the efficiency, effectiveness, and value of health care interventions. The stimulus behind these evaluative efforts is positive: not only is it important to understand which prevention and therapeutic interventions work well, but it is also past time to curb the inflation in health care costs to which our high-tech approach has given impetus.

But something about this shift in orientation from a patient-focused medical approach to one that gives significant weight to communal needs (and communal finances) feels uncomfortable. It has become distressingly obvious that, to more effectively meet the needs of our population, the nation's health care system needs reform. Yet, we still have not been able to "jump in with both feet," discontinue coverage for medical technologies that help only a select few, and direct all of our scarce health care dollars toward health promotion and disease prevention. Our reluctance has little to do with our conviction that change is needed. It has much more to do, I believe, with the epidemiology of hope.

The military recognizes the psychological value of this hope, expending millions of dollars on elaborate systems of transportation and graded health care installations to assure its fighting cadres that if they are injured, everything will be done to save them. Interestingly, public health–oriented interventions have played upon this characteristically American, individualist hope for a second chance. Recall the slogan of a past campaign to encourage people to wear seat belts: "The life you save may be your own."

American people watch with interest and pride as medicine saves the lives of people who appear to be hopelessly ill, rescuing them from the brink of death. The most awesome medical miracles occur in hospitals, but with their steep costs, a growing consensus that we have too many hospital beds, and the movement of health care toward a more population-based, cost-conscious system, the need for so many high-tech and expensive institutions is being questioned. Here the epidemiology of hope arises, muddling the inquiry. Citizens may understand that their city has too many hospitals, but they still may be reluctant to close down the hospital nearest their home. What if they were in an automobile accident and needed trauma care? What if a loved one experienced a massive heart attack? Minutes could mean the difference between life and death.

Americans will not easily yield these institutions to the budgeteer's ax. In all likelihood, we will maintain a more rational sizing and distribution of our hospitals, which will increasingly become almost exclusively large intensive care units. In other words, they will be seen by the public, not incorrectly, as institutions dedicated to bringing people back from the brink of death.

I hope that we citizens will also economize and become much more prudent buyers of such care. We shall all continue to need good professional judgment to make balanced societal allocation decisions between curative and preventive care. To achieve this balance among our mature health care professionals, we need a similar balance in our educational experiences. Although organized medicine and the public health establishment have frequently been at odds, respected professional leaders are working hard to remedy the situation; many are seeking training in both medicine and public health, and, more recently, experimenting with new kinds of educational venues and strategies. Although I believe the "official" gaps will disappear shortly, it will be up to the young people to integrate the two approaches so that each health care professional sees prevention and curing as components of a continuum rather than as irreconcilable competitors.

Chapter Eight

Three Intellectual Paradigms for Both Education and Practice

These days, there are few more overused words than "paradigm." In 1952, a young professor named Thomas Kuhn gave an extended series of lectures in a natural science course I was taking as a college freshman. His lectures became the basis of his famous book, *The Structure of Scientific Revolutions*, and he is the person who introduced the word paradigm to our modern thinking. Kuhn's point was that each scientific era or movement is governed by a theory, or paradigm. This revelation proved fruitful for those who accepted new paradigms and mined them for discoveries. Sometimes, however, when a new paradigm came onto the scene, it was resisted and resented by the establishment. The resulting struggle between paradigms would go on for decades before the new one would finally become dominant. It seems to me appropriate, and even important, to use the word paradigm to describe each of the three major theoretical prisms through which the twenty-first century healer must be able to view the world.

For the past fifty years, physicians have been armed with a growing supply of technical interventions resulting from the nation's investments in basic and applied medical science. This supply has become so pervasive, so effective much of the time, and so alluring both to patients and to practitioners that the profession may have fallen prey to the technologic imperative, losing sight of the healing effect of the physician and nurse as therapies in their own right.

Simply put, the clinician's functions fall into three categories: prevention, cure, and care. Prevention, which implies efforts to help motivate individual patients to adopt healthful lifestyles, also refers to the public health functions of population-wide initiatives. It includes a population-based approach rooted in the science of epidemiology, which I call the Population-Based Public Health Paradigm.

Clearly, some physicians will act more directly than others in promoting health and preventing illness; only a few will dedicate their professional lives to public health. All physicians and other clinicians, however, need to support public health initiatives.

Reductionist Biomedical Paradigm

The modern cure mode, part of what I call the Reductionist Biomedical Paradigm, rests on a disease-focused view, wherein practitioners attempt to understand the molecular defect causing a disease and to determine precise molecular curative interventions. Molecular-level understanding is the building block for the best choice of treatments. The advances in both diagnosis and treatment over the past several decades stagger the imagination. The ongoing genetic revolution promises to yield products and techniques of unlimited promise in terms of both prevention and cure.

Many see this molecular-based, disease-focused paradigm, however, as minimizing the importance of the clinician's interpersonal skills in fostering trust, developing a therapeutic relationship, and facilitating a constructive use of the placebo effect. It underrates the importance of the clinician's ability to deal with patients afflicted by incurable diseases, the suffering that accompanies chronic pain and illness, and the nature and quality of a patient's death and its ramifications for family and friends. In fact, the Reductionist Biomedical Paradigm does not address these issues.

Biopsychosocial Paradigm

The Biopsychosocial Paradigm, clearly espoused by George Engel, provides an intellectual construct that does address these matters. It identifies the disciplines that inform the strategies of human interaction necessary to serve most effectively as the basis for a therapeutic relationship and environment. Engel, Havens, Eisenberg, and Kleinman, among many others, have written extensively about the interface between culture and belief; the interpersonal strategies of the physician; the molecular disease afflicting the person's internal organs; and the healing process afflicting the whole person. This social science–based paradigm leads to the whole-person–oriented interactive skills so critical in helping people cope with illnesses that cannot be cured—skills that are particularly essential in the ongoing care of chronic afflictions.

Linking Two Paradigms With a Third

In recent years, I have sensed that there are growing cadres of young faculty across the spectrum of specialties who perceive medicine more broadly than the older faculty do. Students will probably find the majority of their professors still locked narrowly into one of the paradigms. For example, those faculty most concerned with population-based approaches to reducing the burden of illness on society will tend to scorn as feeble the contribution of much high-tech medicine to improving the societal health status.

Those who do not build bridges between paradigms may be ill-equipped to deliver the best care. For example, psychiatrists and other mental health professionals operating in the Biopsychosocial Paradigm who do not appreciate the benefits of biomedicine and public health risk isolating the mental health enterprise from the rest of the caregiving effort. Similarly, reductionists who fail to respect the theory behind mental health practice only magnify an unnecessary gulf separating "scientific" doctors from psychiatrists and psychologists. In building bridges to other paradigms, the molecularly oriented, technologically based physician should incorporate into the caregiving team people who possess skills from the realm of the Biopsychosocial Paradigm and vice versa.

The Population-Based Public Health Paradigm

One concept that might help both faculty and students bridge the gulf between paradigms is what I described earlier as the epidemiology of hope—that is, the hope that every American holds for revival or repair if disaster strikes. The epidemiology of hope is a societal benefit; many people, including myself, take pride in the amount of resources Americans commit to giving people another chance at life in situations where other societies might abandon them. Single-instance, expensive, reductionist, biomedical therapy that can be applied to only a few appropriate patients has a population-wide benefit: hope for all, should they become afflicted.

Family medicine programs have led the way in creating links among the three paradigms during the past thirty years, in many instances swimming against the

Three Intellectual Paradigms for Health Care

	Population-Based Public Health	Reductionist Biomedical	Biopsychosocial
Conceptual Basis	The health status of the population must be the subject of analysis if we are to measure and understand trends in our people's well-being.	This biomolecular paradigm rests upon the principles of modern reductionism and seeks to identify the molecular basis for disease states and molecular curative interventions.	There is a science to healing humans through human interaction and there are sciences that inform effective communication.
Core Academic Disciplines	Epidemiology Sociology Anthropology Political Science Demography Economics Organization Management	Molecular biology Chemistry Physics Mathematics Physiology Microbiology Immunology Genetics	Psychology Communication Sciences Neuropsychiatry Sociology Anthropology Liberal Arts The Arts
Relative Importance to Prevention, Cure, and Care	Crucial importance to health promotion and disease prevention strategies and research priorities. Important in measuring impact of curative interventions.	Crucial importance to understanding disease and approaches for therapy, forming the bases for many specialties. Of growing importance in prevention (e.g., vaccines and mapping of genetic risks of disease).	Of most importance to the caring mode of medicine, especially in the treatment of chronic disorders, but perhaps having some significance to prevention and health promotion, especially in strategizing.
The Role of the Physician	To promote health and prevent disease by encouraging behavioral change (e.g., nutrition, exercise, vaccination) and attempting to alter risk factors (e.g., smoking, hypertension) before they cause disease. To promote an environment for healthful living. To work constructively on an interprofessional team deployed to deliver necessary and useful preventive and health promotional services.	To focus on the physiologic symptoms of the individual patient and to match treatment regimens with molecular basis of disease in accordance with the best scientific evidence in the context of the patient's situation and desires. To work with other relevant health professionals to ensure efficient delivery of curative services.	To use the interview not only as a tool for collecting objective information and measurements, but also for learning the nature and history of the patient's experiences and clarifying what they mean to the patient as an individual and as a member of society. The integrity of these personal interactions build trust on the part of the patient, enhance compliance with treatment regimens, and promote the placebo effect. To work with others to create a healing team and caring institutions.

reductionist tide of the medical faculty's majority opinion to focus on a more integrative approach to care.

The table on page 84 outlines the disciplines that inform the three paradigms and the techniques and strategies that flow from each of them. Obviously, there is too much here for any formal medical or other health professional educational program to cover. In addition, the role modeling among medical public-health faculty tends to focus exclusively on one of the three paradigms. Students will therefore need to possess an independence of purpose and a stubbornness of spirit to pursue their own broad education as they work to achieve the credentials of a scientifically based healer. The medical student of today should understand, work with, and, as I believe possible, synthesize all three paradigms. Alternatively, physicians who are already working fundamentally within one paradigm should try to achieve a balance of tolerance and respect for the other two.

Crossing bridges between paradigms involves more than just knowledge and technique. There is the matter of commitment to human service. There is also the question about the appropriate perpetuation of a special subset of society to take charge of people's health care and be given extraordinary privilege in return for two things: carrying the torch of hope and the tools of therapy for those who become sick, and initiating the policies and programs that enhance and sustain the population's health status and aim to reduce the overall burden of illness and disease upon the nation.

Are these health professionals doing something special after all? If so, what is their social contract? What do they profess and promise to society? This brings us to the issue of motivation and covenants, discussed in the final section.

IV

The
Need for a
Tenacious
Loyalty

Chapter Nine

Why Become a Caregiver?

N ow we must consider the complex issue of motivation, to which I have previously alluded only briefly. It is a problem that will, and rightly should, haunt aspiring young professionals until they have made the final decision about their practice area.

The wide variety of motivations for entering the health care profession stem from the personal values and interests held by those entering the field. In the end, the variety makes for creative and useful health care career choices that benefit both the patient individually and the public at large. Indeed, health care would still be in the Dark Ages if no physicians had chosen to turn from rendering bedside care to becoming pathologists and laboratory directors. A broad, in-depth medical education is necessary for pathologists and clinical laboratory professionals to facilitate information gathering and diagnostic and therapeutic decision making.

Other specialties of medicine are also highly technologic in nature, requiring little personal interaction with the patient. Radiology, both diagnostic and therapeutic, is an example. In many other areas of specialization—genetic manipulation or laser treatment, for example—necessary scientific skills may quite properly transcend the interpersonal skills required to develop a therapeutic relationship as a potential healer with particular patients. In such instances, the healing lies more in the intervention, treatment, or manipulation and less in the relationship between the particular purveyor of the technology and the patient.

For many decades, Guido Majno, a world-renowned pathologist and biomedical scientist, has maintained a scholarly interest in the history of medicine, and his scholarship and writing reflect as much anthropology as history. In a recent essay, he explores in depth the capacities of previous healers, including the fathers of Western scientific medicine, and contrasts their efforts to those of modern physicians:

> When scientific medicine began to perform its healing miracles (only forty or fifty years ago) there was a marvelous opportunity. Ancient medicine had discovered the secret of helping souls. Now it was possible to help bodies as well, thanks to tons of knowledge, chemicals, and machines. It did not quite work out that way. The new generation of scientific healers was carried away by the physical problems, in fact by anything that could be measured. Spiritual concerns are hard to measure. It was assumed that if the body is healed the rest would somehow follow.
>
> Before long the public began to realize that something was missing. We are now in the midst of a rising anti-medical tide, while scores of supposedly "holistic" would-be do-gooders move in to fill the vacuum. At the latest count there are seventy alternative forms of medicine. They certainly have the secret cure—time—and with it they can offer enough hope and smiles to heal 85 percent of all patients.

Marrying High-Tech and People Skills

Majno questions whether we may have gone wrong by suggesting that the problems begin in medical school: "The old ways are very difficult to teach; nobody yet has found a way to teach the human approach. [It] has [been] said . . . that the human approach 'cannot be taught—although it can be learned.'" In his conclusion, Majno seeks a remedy:

> The message of history, as I have tried to decipher it, is that scientific therapy has eroded the human care which has always been a key part of the healing process. Young medical students, brought up in the system, may find it difficult or impossible to fight the trend. Maybe so, but there is hope. Awareness of the problem is a first step toward solving it. . . . It may be impossible to stretch minutes into hours, but the quality of those minutes can certainly be improved.

Majno believes that turning to the lessons of past masters of Western medicine and other forms of healing can help physicians learn how to use the diminished time available to them to convey their concern and attentiveness to the patient's suffering. Through the marriage of humanity with the growing supply of scientific interventions, Majno anticipates that today's physicians can reverse the current antimedical trend and become the most powerful healers the world has ever known.

The difficulty with the many kinds of motivation that people bring to the practice of medicine lies in finding a proper balance between a desire to provide direct human service and a need to master a wide variety of sciences and technologies before being recognized as a physician. Without maintaining scientific knowledge and technical competence throughout one's professional lifetime, all the good will in the world can provide only less than optimal care. Alternatively, for those physicians daily involved with the provision of highly personal health services, high technical competence without the people skills necessary to build trust and confidence also leads to far less than the optimal state we seek for our patients.

The Desire to Win

Let us highlight just briefly the differing motivations that bring scientists into their respective fields. I recall being troubled occasionally by the high degree of competitiveness among elite scientists. There is a sometimes pervasive element of seeking, let's say, the Nobel Prize, the brass ring, or the financial gain for discovering some fantastically useful new tool. More common, perhaps, the scientist is driven by the fun of the pursuit and the challenge of the intellectual problem, rather than by a need to serve suffering humanity.

Tracy Thompson, a writer who says her life was dramatically improved by the drug Prozac, has eloquently described her pursuit of the creators of this drug. She wanted to understand why they created it and what they felt after reaching their goal. Bryan Molloy of Lilly Research Labs was the primary scientist of the three inventors of the new drug. Molloy stunned Thompson with his answer to her question, "How does it make you feel to know that what you have done has helped people—to know that this molecule you invented has allowed me to live my life in a way I never thought possible?" Molloy replied:

> This puts me in a somewhat embarrassing position. . . . The company puts itself in the position of saying it is here to help people, and I'm here saying I didn't do it for that. I just wanted to do it for the intellectual high. It looked like scientific fun.

The Desire to Heal

Compare Molloy's motivation with what must have been at the root of the efforts of Edward L. Trudeau, a physician and clinical investigator who became best known for his leadership in establishing the premier American sanitarium for tuberculosis patients (in the Adirondack mountains of New York). Trudeau contracted tuberculosis in 1873, when it was believed that the disease was uniformly fatal and either inherited or due to some perverted humor or spiritual problem. It was not thought to be infectious.

In 1887, Trudeau undertook a starkly simple and elegant experiment; the results convinced him of the need for fresh air, good nutrition, and ample rest when treating tuberculosis. The experiment involved fifteen rabbits, divided equally into three treatment groups. The rabbits in the first group were injected with a standard inoculum of tubercle bacilli; they were then placed on an island (with no other rabbits) on which they could forage comfortably. One of these rabbits died of the disease; the other four returned to normal life after fibrosis of the initial lesion. The rabbits in the second group were also injected with tubercle bacilli, but were kept in a cage in a dark cellar with minimal nutrition. All five died of tuberculosis. The control group, which did not get injected with tubercle bacilli, was placed in the cellar with the same poor food as the second group. No animals from the control group died, although all lost weight on the regimen.

Trudeau's science, at least in the case of this experiment, arose out of an interest to seek a cure for a generally fatal disease with which he was also afflicted. His motivation was in a different category than the quest for honor, fortune, or intellectual achievement.

The Desire to Serve

An old aphorism, which I find overly simplistic, holds that there are two kinds of people in the world: those who use people and those who serve people. My discomfort with the aphorism is abated, however, if I add a third category to which I find that most other people (including me) belong: those who sometimes use people and sometimes serve people.

Within this third category is a distinction between those people who wish they served others more or all of the time, and those who really prefer to use others more often and more effectively than they currently do. Where do you stand with relation to these categories?

I have always felt that for serious caregivers, the concept of service must achieve a status akin to a secular sacrament that transcends the benevolent self-interest of the businessperson to please the customer in all matters. Service is surely good "business" for the caregiver, but it is also something more fundamental than customer relations efforts for both the caregiver and the care recipient. A customer's need for satisfaction from an automobile dealer, for instance, pales in comparison to the needs and satisfaction of a customer—the patient— in a health care setting, in which the patient requires a businessperson—the caregiver—in whom they can completely trust with matters of grave personal importance (if not life and death).

In the middle of this century, the philosopher Gabriel Marcel mourned the debasement of the concept of service in the modern, bureaucratic, egalitarian state. He saw service to other human beings as the most fundamental, if not the highest, human activity. Marcel was troubled that in our increasingly bureaucratic society the typical citizen felt that he or she owed to others only the minimum standard of service as delineated in a contract—that much and no more—and was less often governed by an actual covenant between two people than by the laws or mores of society.

It is instructive to think of his arguments, made many decades ago, in the context of the modern systems of managed care with their heavy institutional, and hence bureaucratic, overlay of values and procedures regarding the provision of service.

In *The Call of Service—A Witness to Idealism*, Robert Coles, a physician, psychiatrist, and social critic, relates several stories about people he has found who have made a unique commitment to service. He makes an important distinction when he describes his understanding of the differing personal foundational positions taken by his mother and his father with relation to service. Coles, himself a service devotee, finds his parents' approaches equally valid and meaningful.

He describes his mother as a deeply religious person with a lifelong commitment to understanding her motivations and to trying to orient herself and her life to providing service to other people. She created an explicit tie between her daily activities, her philosophy of living, and her religion. His father, on the other hand, is described as someone who dedicated himself to serving others later in life and who seldom articulated his reasons for doing so, being both rather pragmatic ("Just do it!") and somewhat circumspect about what he might find if he probed too far into his deepest motives.

Coles describes his encounter in the 1950s with Thomas Merton, a contemplative monk and writer, and attempts to analyze the nature of the healing impact the monk had on him and others. In Coles's view, Merton's power as a healer arose from the fact that Merton had known and continued to know personal suffering.

He was able to draw out the most painful problems from others, because they could perceive that he personally shared in and understood their suffering.

Of course, all of us have our burdens; Merton's gift came from being able to transmit both a sense of his own encounters with difficulty and a nonjudgmental acceptance of other people, whatever their difficulties. Through the story of Merton, Coles presents his readers with the strange paradox of a contemplative monk who had retreated from the world but was continuously sought out in person and through letters by a wide variety of suffering people. Remarkably, he somehow was effective in ministering to many of them. According to Coles,

> Dorothy Day and Daniel Berrigan and Walker Percy and so many others sought Merton out. I especially remember Dorothy Day's remarks about him: "He had known much pain, and he knew how to lift pain from others." She was content to state those two aspects of Merton without connecting the one to the other in what people like me call a psychodynamic way. Nevertheless, she knew that an essential and important part of Merton's life was his passionate desire to minister unto others, to hear from them, learn of their tensions and turmoil, and tell them of his, too. Once Dorothy Day said this about Merton as we talked of his voluminous writing: "He cured with words—all the time he did! I know! I can remember those letters, the good medicine they were to me. And I always knew that with Merton it was the doctor healing himself as well as the rest of us who were his patients."

Coles goes on to describe Merton's impact on a stranger:

> Merton . . . venture[d] to Asia, ever anxious to be connected with wisdom and with healing other than the kind he knew. . . . A person present at the conference . . . remarked upon his kindly manner, the gentleness he radiated and its calming effect on her: to the very last that humane touch of grace offered without guile or pretense to others.

The Service Ethic Versus the Power Ethic

It may well be that the most important insight I received into the meaning of the service gestalt came when I left the world of doctoring for full-time participation in the world of administering. It took the soul-numbing experience of being an activist administrator to make me appreciate that the world of administration cannot be handled with a service mentality alone. One also needs commitment to some vision of a better future.

My wife and I discovered this when some unpopular decisions I had made prompted anonymous death threats to my wife and me and sinister threats of abduction of our young daughters. An almost daily escalation of this sort of activity, designed to force us to give up and leave town, made our lives miserable. Yet, like most people faced with such a prospect, we recognized that little is gained by giving up, and perhaps all is lost if one yields to the pressure to run.

We decided to stay, but nonetheless discovered that the dread and angst did not go away with each new dawn. Instead, each day merely reminded me that we seemed to be locked in a power struggle with intelligent people operating under a different philosophy, resulting in a serious game of cat and mouse. One day as my wife and I drove to work, we developed a strategy that seemed to strengthen and satisfy us; it was a strategy that also returned us to our service foundations. Each morning, as we mused about what dreadful things might happen to us during the ensuing day, we concluded that we should each decide on one person for whom we would do something positive that day, and report the result back to each other on the way home that evening.

We found that our joy in living returned, our capacity to deal with a hostile environment grew by leaps and bounds, our sense of satisfaction and personal meaning was made whole, and our essentially positive and constructive perception of the world and our place in it was reestablished. We discovered the strength to stay the course and overcome our difficulties.

Tension Between the Service Ethic and the Ethos of 'Scientific' Clinical Practice

One of the best articulations of the divergent pulls on the physician of patient care and the science of medicine appears in Sherwin Nuland's *How We Die: Reflections on Life's Final Chapter.* As I discussed in chapter 6, the drive to solve The Riddle brings physicians into direct conflict with the best interests of some of their patients for whom The Riddle may be of no concern. The Riddle, for Nuland and the young doctors growing to professional maturity over the past four decades, relates to the drive to determine what is happening at the molecular level, primarily because such a discovery may lead to a cure. A dogged pursuit of the answers to The Riddle, however, may not always be what the patient wants. The patient, for example, may be in the process of dying and may prefer help with an easier death, rather than an overabundance of costly, high-tech hindrances to a peaceful passing. I recommend Dr. Nuland's book to all beginning practitioners because it describes a real-life situation that every experienced physician and other clinician has inevitably encountered, one with which we all must deal: the process of dying.

Meanwhile, it seems useful to share briefly with you the thoughts of Lewis Thomas, America's famous physician-scientist turned literary figure and popular philosopher. In an interview from his deathbed, Thomas, the consummate devotee of the evolution of living species, seemed to say that the human species is intrinsically good at being useful:

> If we paid more attention to this biological attribute, we'd get a satisfaction that cannot be attained from goods or knowledge. If you can contemplate the times when you've been useful, even indispensable, to other people, the review of our lives would begin to have effects on the younger generations. . . . Plain usefulness.

Because medical science will constitute so much of the education of aspiring professionals, and because biomedical scientists may predominate among their early (and perhaps later) role models, students will be exposed to all of the attitudes and values associated with service and usefulness. They may well find it challenging to harmonize the primary motivations of scientists with the primary motivations of a clinician-caregiver.

A Personal, Simplistic View of Service and Physicianhood

My view of the central motivating characteristic of someone in the direct caregiving professions became clear to me in a recent episode that involved my barber. He is a naturalized citizen who combines great common sense and cynicism about the world with an instinct that tells him he should stay away from doctors and medicine if at all possible. One day, I observed that he was limping and commented on it. He explained that his right foot had just begun to hurt and that he was sure it would go away soon. He didn't want to talk about any medications.

Two weeks later, when I made my next visit to the shop, my barber was obviously still in considerable distress from his sore foot. He volunteered that he was thinking about giving up active barbering and running his business from his desk. When I asked, he told me he had not seen a doctor, had no intention of doing so, and had taken no medication. He did permit me to examine his foot, however, whereupon I quickly determined that the most likely problem was an acute tendinitis. I suggested that he might get tremendous relief from some readily available medications.

His response made it clear to me that he was unlikely to get the medicine and that the best way for me to achieve compliance from this nonpatient was to walk the two blocks to the pharmacy, pick up the medicine, and deliver it to him personally. He was certainly surprised when I returned to the shop, remedies in hand.

The next morning on my way to work, I stopped by to see how the medication had worked. My barber reported that he was pain-free and again registered surprise that a doctor was going to all this effort at no charge to him. He has been well ever since and has even taken a few precautions to protect against a recurrence. He has been cured completely, or so he believes, and it made me happy to have made some good guesses about how to help him get relief.

As for myself, I was surprised that my sense of satisfaction at a simple and routine intervention in a commonplace disorder was every bit as great as at any of those rare moments in medicine when one deciphers a complex problem and solves a therapeutic riddle. From the patient's perspective, a nettlesome problem had been solved. It did not matter how simple or demanding the intellectual or technical intervention required of the physician to achieve the solution. I was in fact, by nature, a physician.

I conclude that caregiving health professionals are likely to be happiest in their profession if, in fact, helping others gives them real satisfaction. Do you like to hold doors open for others to pass through, or do you prefer to have others hold doors for you? Would you like to develop a healing presence or personality as described in Coles's essay on Merton? Or would you rather prescribe a pill and move on to the next case?

Although these questions are simplistic, and although the most tangible indices of service orientation are different for each person, they point to the importance of bringing honesty and careful self-reflection to selecting a career at which you can work both effectively and happily.

A New Service Ethic: Collaboration

People just entering the profession of medicine face a new challenge, or an old challenge with a new and expanding dimension. By this I refer to the growing number of professionals on the health care delivery team and the increasing complexity of the health care delivery system. It is no longer simply patient and doctor; today, it is the patient and literally hundreds of members of the health care team. Teamwork is being brought to bear on the problems of individual patients within the context of the entire population's needs and health status. One physician's dedication to serve a patient is no longer sufficient to achieve the desired outcome. Instead, we must learn to collaborate across professions in the patient's best interests.

This collaboration must occur at the bedside and consultation room levels, as well as at the juncture where institutional and organizational ethics and values come together. This imperative, taking on a heightened importance, is not new because we have always had to work in teams. The current environment, however, makes collaboration critical to success; those who cannot collaborate will not be as successful in the final analysis.

For good and for bad, the impact of institutional values on individual values and behaviors, along with the interplay between individual and organizational ethics, will become increasingly important to health care delivery. Service-oriented and service-driven professionals will want to be continuously involved in shaping both the interplay of professionals on the team and the organized systems within which the team works. There are techniques available to enhance collaboration, and satisfactions arise from successful collaboration. I hold that the commitment to help and the drive to excellence in professional service must now also include the drive to collaborate successfully with others who can enhance clinical outcomes. Thus, to those tenets of competence and caring that have guided physician practice since Hippocrates, we must now add *collaboration*.

Chapter Ten

Commitment and Healing

Excerpts from the Physician's Oath by Hippocrates

I will look upon him who shall have taught me this art even as one of my parents. I will share my substance with him, and I will supply his necessities, if he be in need. I will regard his offspring even as my own brethren and I will teach them this art, if they would learn it without fee or covenant. I will impart this art by precept, by lecture and by every mode of teaching, not only to my own sons but to sons of him who has taught me, and to disciples bound by covenant and oath, according to the law of medicine.

The regimen I adopt shall be for the benefit of my patients according to my ability and judgment, and not for their hurt or for any wrong. I will give no deadly drug to any, though it be asked of me, nor will I counsel such, and especially I will not aid a woman to procure abortion. Whatsoever house I enter, there will I go for the benefit of the sick, refraining from all wrongdoing or corruption, and especially from any act of seduction of male or female, of bond or free. Whatsoever things I see or hear concerning the life of men, in my attendance on the sick or even apart therefrom, which ought not to be noised abroad, I will keep silence thereon, counting such things to be as sacred secrets.

So reads the portion of the Physician's Oath that generations of medical students have taken upon graduation from medical school. This distillation of the teachings of the "father of medicine" has endured for a remarkable period of time; it was recorded around 400 B.C.! In fact, the beginning of the oath calls on

Apollo Physician, Asclepius, Health, Panacea, and all of the gods and goddesses to serve as witness to the words that follow within the oath. Although historians largely agree that the oath was written not by Hippocrates but by his followers after his death, the oath is consistent with the distinctive combination of humanistic concern and practical wisdom that appears in the writing of Hippocrates, an emphasis that has inspired and guided many a physician.

Precepts to Cherish or Question

Although Hippocrates probably did not construct the Physician's Oath, it affords some insight into the "person" Hippocrates. To me, the meaning of the Hippocratic oath and the reason for its enduring value is its highly personal quality, reflecting the basic concept of devotion to people and a desire to serve them.

Upon careful study, the oath offers much wisdom, even for modern-day physicians. It is clear, however, that it contains some statements that do not reflect the beliefs held by many twentieth-century physicians. Scholars have noted that, in light of current knowledge and the needs of this century, the oath could be improved with reinterpretation. It no longer seems to capture all the responsibilities and obligations of physicians.

Medicine has become enormously complex; consequently, today's modern physicians not only practice general patient care, but serve as highly trained specialists, research scientists, full-time teachers, or administrators concerned with medical education, delivering health care services, or organizing our vast biomedical research efforts. Comments physician and ethicist Edmund Pellegrino:

> In a simpler world, that [Hippocratic] ethic long sufficed to guide the physician in his service to patient and community. Today, the intersection of medicine with contemporary science, technology, social organization, and changed human values have revealed significant missing dimensions in the ancient ethic.

Medical Training—Who and How

Among the aspects of the Physician's Oath that many say are outdated are its tenets about medical training and eligibility to join the profession. The oath holds that doctors should teach medicine to their sons, to the sons of their teachers, and to other disciples choosing to live by the "law of medicine." Of course, as more and more women join the health care field, the male bias of the Physician's Oath is no longer appropriate. And, given the intricacy of modern medicine, teaching by apprenticeship or discipleship is no longer feasible. As physician John Leversee notes, health science educators and planners have greatly broadened the kinds of training they look for in candidates for medical school and in the field.

Delivering Care—Who and How

The need to expand the number and kinds of persons involved in delivering health care today is clear. Not only have the numbers of health care professionals increased, but new kinds of professionals—such as occupational therapists, respiratory therapists, nurse practitioners, and radiologic technicians—have taken on unique roles. Technological developments and changing health care needs have made it necessary to train nonphysician professionals in broader skills and responsibilities. No longer is it a particular advantage to be a son of a doctor or a teacher of medicine. Motivation and performance are more important than legacy for gaining entry to education in the health professions.

New Ethical Considerations

Several other circumstances have drawn modern medicine away from its Hippocratic traditions. There is a need to expand our understanding of the ethics of medicine. Biomedical research involving human subjects, for example, challenges the idea that physicians may use only their skills to benefit those in their care. The notion of the physician as a benevolent and paternalistic figure who makes all the decisions for the patient is inconsistent with today's notion of the educated health care consumer. Informed consent was not an issue in Hippocrates' time. Changes in public and medical attitudes about abortion and euthanasia could also make it difficult for today's physician to honor the portions of the oath that proscribe these procedures.

New Social Responsibilities

Still others have argued that the most important reason to update the Physician's Oath is its lack of attention to the responsibilities of the medical profession as a whole. The tension between the interests of the individual and those of the community is not acknowledged in the oath, which focuses exclusively on the responsibilities of physicians to individual patients. Pellegrino comments on the significance of the notion of communal responsibility:

> Society supports the doctor in the expectation that he will direct himself to socially relevant health problems, not just those he finds interesting or remunerative. The commitment to social egalitarianism demands a greater sensitivity to social ethics than is to be found in traditional codes.

William F. May agrees with Pellegrino. In *The Physician's Covenant: Images of the Healer in Medical Ethics*, May describes several images that capture the ways in which society perceives the physician (and in which physicians may perceive themselves). One image is what May calls the "covenanter." As covenanter, the physician has a debt to society for his or her education; he or she also has a debt to patients, who provide a kind of education for the doctor who "practices" on them. In return for public support and public trust, the physician as covenanter reciprocates with service, fidelity, accountability, and responsibility for distribution of basic services. Each of May's images of the healer provides a fascinating window on the roles and

William F. May's Images of the Healer

Fighter   The healer is a fighter against death, battling such enemies as cancer and heart attacks. Patients prize a kind of military intelligence, tactical brilliance, self-confidence, and stamina in the healer. The language of war dominates the understanding of disease (e.g., cancer "invades," the heart suffers an "attack") and shapes the healer's response (e.g., searching for a magic "bullet," utilizing an "armamentarium" of drugs).

Parent   The healer's role is to nurture and reassure patients and shelter them from the powers that are harming them. Kindness rather than candor is the chief moral virtue expected of the healer. As between parent and child, the healer's relationship with the patient is characterized by compassion (e.g., shared suffering) and self-expenditure (i.e., the imbalance of knowledge and power define the healer as the giver and the patient as the receiver).

Technician   Excellent technical performance becomes the effective center of the professional ethic; the healer finds satisfaction in service, but technology and technical performance supply his or her ultimate justification. The healer's white lab coat points to the scientific origin of medical authority and hints at the body mechanic at work. The criteria for admission to medical school and the grading system that prevails there emphasize the preeminent place of technical performance in the formation and career of the professional.

Covenanter   Healers have distinctive obligations to their patients and to their teachers (as in the Hippocratic oath). Patients effectively "teach" healers by allowing healers to "practice" on them. Healers also owe a debt to the society that supports their training; they owe competence, accountability, the courage to hold fellow professionals accountable, and responsibility for the distribution of basic services. Service and fidelity are chief moral virtues of the healer. The patient is a bonded partner in pursuit of health.

Teacher   The healer respects patients' intelligence and power of self-determination. To be an effective teacher requires a kind of imagination that permits the healer to enter into the life circumstances of the patient/learner to reckon with the difficulties the patient faces in acquiring, assimilating, and acting on what he or she needs to know. These skills are particularly important in preventive, rehabilitative, chronic, and terminal care; they often go unrewarded in third-party payment systems and receive little attention in medical schools and residency programs.

responsibilities of the healer. I heartily recommend his book to all of those, whether just entering or well-established, in the healing professions.

Pellegrino agrees with May that physicians have a covenantal relationship with society and cannot absolve themselves from responsibility for deficiencies in distribution, quality, and accessibility of care to the poor and disenfranchised. These defects, widespread today, are examples of the kinds of situations that the Physician's Oath, even with its ethical sensibilities and high moral tone, is insufficient to address.

The Durability of the Ancient Oath

How, despite its jagged-edged fit with modern medicine, does the Physician's Oath endure? Although several attempts have been made to create new oaths that convey the current context for medicine, most graduating medical students still prefer to take the ancient oath. Perhaps it is because they can thereby make a spiritual link with the fascinating, almost magical, world of ancient Greece. Or perhaps reciting the oath connects them in some way to the 2,500-year-old roots of Western scientific medicine, to the prestige of a select group, or to history. In brief, the oath allows the new physician to become part of a tradition that transcends personal interests and rivets attention on superordinate goals.

Certainly, the oath has persisted because of its core premises: competence, commitment, and caring, those foundational values that remain at the heart of modern physicianhood. A few years ago, however, I made my own attempt to fashion a revised version of the Hippocratic oath; it harkens back to some of the enduring and fundamental qualities of the original while integrating some realities of modern life. I firmly believe that, today more than ever, a modern Hippocrates and the Hippocratic profession need a compelling and meaningful covenant to guide activities that otherwise promise to become even more complex, bureaucratic, and impersonal.

The Oath of the Modern Hippocrates

By all that I hold highest, I promise my patients competence, integrity, candor, personal commitment to their best interests, compassion, and absolute discretion and confidentiality within the law.

I shall do by my patients as I would be done by, shall obtain consultation whenever I or they desire, shall include them to the extent they wish in all impor-

tant decisions, and shall minimize suffering whenever a cure cannot be obtained, understanding that a dignified death is an important goal in everyone's life.

I shall try to establish a friendly relationship with my patients and shall accept each one in a nonjudgmental manner, appreciating the validity and worth of different value systems and according to each person a full measure of human dignity.

I shall charge only for my professional services and shall not profit financially in any other way as a result of the advice and care I render my patients.

I shall not accept financial or other incentives as a reward for restricting patient access to medically needed diagnosis or treatment.

I shall provide advice and encouragement for my clients in their efforts to sustain their own health.

I shall work with my profession to improve the quality of medical care and to improve the public health, but I shall not let any lesser public or professional consideration interfere with my primary commitment to provide the best and most appropriate care available to each of my patients.

To the extent that I live by these precepts, I shall be a worthy physician.

Covenant for Collaboration

In the relatively short time since I drafted the above oath, there has arisen even greater recognition of the value (and in many cases, the necessity) of health care professionals delivering care in teams. The personal commitment of the physician to the patient was sufficient when the medical team averaged one doctor and three other professionals. However, the health care team has expanded to include over 120 distinct health professionals. (Not counted are the variety of other people who have a role in health care decision making, including health system administrators, third-party payers, and patients and their families.) Collaboration has taken on an importance of which Hippocrates never dreamt.

Thus, no modern covenant for health care professionals would be complete without acknowledging the need for collaboration among the members of the health care team. In the complicated and sometimes perplexing arena of health care, only groups of professionals who function as a caring and competent team can deliver high quality, highly effective care. In acknowledgment of the importance of collaboration, some colleagues and I have developed a health professions covenant for our times that could supplement the individual oaths taken by graduates of each of the health professions.

A Health Professions Covenant for Our Time

As a health care professional dedicated to enhancing the health care needs and well-being of individuals and communities, I pledge collaboration with all of my health professional colleagues similarly committed, and promise to place the patient's and the public's interests above the self-interests of my individual profession.

Fulfillment of the more traditional tenets of health care espoused by the ancient Hippocratic oath—competence, commitment, and caring—increasingly depends on collaboration. It is my hope that health professionals consider incorporating such a statement into the covenantal ceremonies preceding their entry into the world of practice.

Institutional Values and Commitment

Most people spend the majority of their waking hours within larger institutions—at work or at school, for example. Our society is only now beginning to appreciate how an institution's values can have far-reaching effects. For example, an institution that declares its mission to be improving the health of the community undermines its credibility and commitment when it does not take tangible steps to improve the health of its own employees (for example, through anti–cigarette smoking and anti–substance abuse campaigns, or through diet and exercise programs), who are expected to carry out its mission.

Health care institutions that place excessive value on the number of patient visits their professionals accumulate, the number of dollars saved or dollars earned, and other economic goals run the risk of compromising care by placing too many constraints on the professionals. When rationing technology and, perhaps more significantly, time characterize an institution's mores, commitment to serving patients and collaboration in meeting patient needs are jeopardized.

A revealing perspective on institutional values about the use of time emerges from a 1973 study of senior divinity students at Princeton University. The authors, psychologists John Darley and C. Daniel Batson, contrived an elaborate experiment to study people's capacity to help someone in need. (It would not be permitted today because it involved deceiving the subjects.)

Near the end of the semester, the divinity students were to meet individually with an instructor on a topic. A portion of the students was instructed to talk about the parable of the Good Samaritan; the other students were asked to discuss suitable jobs or professions for seminary students. Students were given a few minutes to prepare, after which time the staff assistant returned with instructions for going to an adjacent building to deliver the talk to the instructor. The students were informed of one of three time constraints:

- "Hurry, you're already late." (the "hurried" group)
- "They're ready for you now—please go right over." (the "somewhat hurried" group)
- "It will be a few minutes before they're ready for you, but you'd best head over." (the "unhurried" group)

On the way to the adjacent building to present the talk, each student encountered a young man writhing on the ground in pain. He was actually a paid, trained observer playing the modern counterpart of the sufferer encountered by the Good Samaritan. His job was to record which students stopped, what they did when they stopped, and how long they stayed.

When the data were analyzed, the only variable that correlated with whether a student stopped to offer assistance was the time available before the student was expected to arrive. Of the group as a whole, 40 percent offered some form of aid to the man in pain. When evaluated against time constraints, 63 percent in the "unhurried" group, 45 percent in the "somewhat hurried" group, and only 10 percent in the "hurried" group stopped to help. There was no escaping the conclusion, wrote the authors, that the decision to care for a person in distress was predominantly a function of having the time to do so. Put another way, even those with the very best intentions require time to be of help to a suffering person.

This tragic choice between time and caring is made every day in our nation's hospitals, health clinics, and doctors' offices. What we know about the placebo effect, taking care of those who are suffering, staying by those who are facing death, and the healing power of words tells us that rationing time could have dire consequences, at least, for patients. As we work to make the health care system more cost-effective, we recognize that reducing the time spent with a patient and, along with it, the tools of communication, companionship, compassion, and shared decision making may indeed reduce costs. But doing so will also dramatically compromise value, and may prove disastrous to the whole of medicine. It will undermine the healing relationship between health care professionals and patients, as well as between institutions and patients.

As we move toward utilizing large and complex not-for-profit organized delivery systems based upon prepaid, capitated financial arrangements, the traditional covenantal understanding between patient and physician could be dramatically affected. If the dual objectives of patient autonomy and empowerment and physician advocacy for the patient's best interests are to be sustained within these organized delivery systems, then it is clear that these systems and corporate entities will have to agree to an institutional ethic that supports these ethical priorities for patients and physicians. Law professor and ethicist Susan Wolf has presented a recent detailed review that demonstrates the criticality of the issue of institutional ethics and their developing impact on physician ethics.

How might institutions, ranging from small clinics and community hospitals to massive academic health centers, approach the concept of institutional ethics? Health policy expert David Mechanic notes that, to counter the erosion of public trust in various elements of our health care system, medical institutions are conducting public information programs, seeking feedback from patient-consumers, and educating their staffs to become more responsive and culturally sensitive. Mechanic also comments on the initiatives designed to empower patients further:

> These range across preventive health programs, family planning, pregnancy and childbirth, women's health, and chronic disease programs. At the social level, health institutions are more likely to put patient representatives on their boards and committees. In some long-term patient services, the patients themselves or family members may participate in certain recruiting or hiring decisions. Moreover, it is not uncommon for client groups themselves to organize and administer services, as exemplified in some programs for persons with disabilities.

Some institutions have developed formal institutional covenants. For example, with the help of an ethicist, M.D. Anderson Cancer Center in Houston has created a patient-based code of care. Edmund Pellegrino emphasizes that people not involved in health care professions must be included among the drafters of institutional covenants. Other institutions could, and perhaps should, follow suit.

Two sayings derived from religious writings, when transformed into the health care vernacular, may serve to summarize some of the key personal and institutional values that I advocate here. The first is St. Paul's: "There are faith, hope and charity! These three! And the greatest of these is charity!" The health care version might be as follows: "There are prevention, curing, and caring! These three! And the greatest of these is caring!"

The second saying is: "God is first; everyone else is second; and I am third!" This epigram could become: "The patients (and the public) are first; the profession is second; and I am third!"

It is crucial for the next generation of physicians and other caregivers to continually reexamine the validity and cultural and personal meaning of an oath or covenant. The alternative is contractual health care that carefully delineates what and how much will be done in exchange for what and how much—and no more! If, in fact, there is any validity to the central theme of this book—that our health care enterprise exists to provide competent and caring intervention to suffering people—then it clearly follows that clinicians covenanted to that role are best suited to provide patients with satisfaction in their quest for mercy.

Postscript

When she read the penultimate form of this manuscript, a friend and experienced clinician-educator commented that she was left with one unanswered question, a question that she confronts with increasing frequency in her interactions with medical students and generalist physicians in postgraduate training. She indicated that she deemed my manuscript incomplete without at least attempting to address this question. Many members of the young, up-and-coming generation of clinicians, she explained, are asking, "If we are to internalize this commitment to service, to focus primarily on the sufferings of others, and to adhere to the primary ethical precept of competence based upon the latest science and the latest technology with a large dose of psychology and sociology thrown in, how can we be fair to our spouses and children and do our share as friends, neighbors, and members of the community?" They wonder, "Aren't we allowed some time for our recreation and personal development? In brief, how can we have—or get—a life?"

At first, I believed that I couldn't even attempt a response, partly because I am at the other end of the professional and personal trails and perhaps can't adequately place myself in their shoes. Mostly, however, I hesitated to respond because I am a biased observer whose views should be somewhat suspect for the young. After all, I currently am not a practicing clinician. More important, I grew up in what I think of as the Vince Lombardi era of medicine, an era in which admission to medical school presumed that one had the physical and mental strength and durability sufficient to endure the most rigorous training—training to prepare for the most serious of situations. The atmosphere that prevailed can be likened to both the benefits and the drawbacks of the well-known Green Bay Packers championship football teams coached by the legendary Vince Lombardi. In football, this male-dominated, driven environment produced spectacular victories, but at what personal sacrifice? In medicine, the Lombardi era was one in which very few students were married during medical school (because they might lose their single-minded focus); in which only five to seven percent of incoming medical school classes were women; in which many of the best residency programs in surgery, medicine, and some other specialties involved living in the hospital (with explicit and implicit encouragement not to marry); and in which the standard operating routine during the three to five years of postgraduate hospital-based training was to be on duty in the hospital every other night and every other weekend. Having survived and benefited from that educational environment, I have been shaped by it as well, and therefore I should remain removed from any effort to translate the values of the clinical professions to the current age for the upcoming generation of healers.

My friend still wasn't satisfied, however, after hearing my defense. Upon reflection, my reticence to address the question, though well founded, now strikes me as something of a cop-out; I know from personal experience that her students' question is one that I hear frequently. Although I am aware that my answer may be unsatisfying to some, here it is.

First, if becoming a committed and competent scientific healer is your professional goal, you must challenge yourself to accomplish that in conjunction with your other goals as a person with family and civic responsibilities. You have a constellation of personal and professional objectives, which may be one of your major generational contributions to the health professions. Second, you must realize that it is virtually impossible to accomplish this alone, as a professional single-handedly in charge of the delivery of health care services to a panel of patients or to a population; you must work with others in a team or group with the same general values and aims. With these realities in mind, we are in the midst of a huge transition to implement various forms of health care service. There is no escaping that many of these forms are grossly inadequate, sometimes fatally flawed, and occasionally marred by human venality accompanying altered financial incentives to get rich in the business.

There may always be the Vince Lombardis in our professions who can productively give 110 percent of themselves to the care of the sick. We should celebrate them. We must celebrate equally the new road that the rest of us must find to achieve a balance between personal and professional goals. Women physicians are leading us toward that balance, because they, in particular, are insisting on being fair to their children and their families. As we all know, that insistence should be shared by men physicians, who (married or not) need to realize that they, too, must be able to participate fully in the lives of their families and their communities.

In sharp contrast to my current way of thinking, in my early professional days I honestly believed that I was so committed and involved with care of the sick that I owed absolutely nothing to any other aspect of society. In addition, I was so underpaid and so lacking in funds that I deemed myself clearly excused from making any financial contribution to any community efforts, whether it be my college, church, or the United Way. I must admit that that frame of mind persisted well beyond the time when I was so busy and so financially challenged. The fact that people like me are still in leadership roles in many of our institutions, programs, and organizations thus proves to be a major difficulty for young clinicians today.

The world of practice is evolving, however. We are, in the truest sense, all in this together. The older generation must adjust as rapidly and effectively as it can, without losing sight of the core values of the enterprise (which are what I have tried to address in this book). More importantly, the younger generation must lead us in the changes for the next millennium, trying (I hope) to sort out and preserve the core values of the past.

It seems to me that all health professionals, and physicians in particular (as the "high priests" of scientific medicine), should reflect on the danger of being perceived as being too removed from the interests of the average citizen—as being too elitist and therefore open to the charge of arrogance. Our professional culture often bases its drive to excel on such a committed single-mindedness that family lives are compromised, spouses are ignored, and children grow up not knowing their parent. As a result a message of contradiction, paradox, and falsehood is sent to a watching public. The message says that this elite profession, to whose members society transfers much wealth and accords much status because of their commitment to alleviating human suffering, actually in its professional workings runs over people and sometimes destroys lives. Health professionals must be certain that human values are expressed in our profession and in our interactions with the people we serve. Thus, we need to reshape our professional lives to allow our clinicians the flexibility to have healthy families and participate more fully in the community at large. If we do not do so, we will hurt the health professions in the long run.

We look forward to these new adjustments, but it is true that younger professionals need help now, tomorrow, or next week; therefore, there must be people to whom to turn for advice regarding this interface between professional and personal development. Clearly, for clinicians, these persons should include our professional mentors—people to whom, all too often, mentees are overly reticent to turn. It is true that such an approach could be poorly handled or disregarded by an inadequate mentor; but you may be surprised at the constructive and thoughtful responses that such queries elicit.

Upon reflection, I realize that I have had many mentors who, in the aggregate, have helped me profoundly. One of my experiences is particularly relevant to discuss here. As I was completing my last year of medical training, I was offered three job opportunities in three parts of the country, each with different basic characteristics and different prospects for my wife's professional future as a basic medical scientist. I laid all of this out in great detail in a multipaged epistle to one of my clinical mentors (who, at the time, was 3,000 miles away) and asked him for advice on making the choice. He was a medical leader with an accomplished wife and a full and well-developed family life.

I got back a characteristically terse and incisive one sentence answer, which went something like this: "Dear Roger, In my experience, decisions like this are periumbilical rather than supratentorial. Good luck. Sincerely."

That advice, delivered in such a simple and direct way, had a great impact on me and on us as a couple. It somehow empowered us to think about what was best for our collective future; it helped me to put rational analysis in its proper place. My mentor's reference to gut feeling, to intuition, was shorthand for placing one's professional life in the perspective of the more holistic concerns of family, environment, and background.

If our professional worlds have become bigger and seem more impersonal than they once might have been, we need not hesitate to seek advice and assistance from others more experienced regarding some of the important personal challenges we face.

One of the next generation's major contributions will be to establish the necessity of a balanced life even as its members achieve heightened capacities to treat disease, heal people, and promote health. As you, in this rising group, attempt to balance your legitimate goals and the mores of the past in a shifting health care environment, you will likely have a difficult time working it all out. But only you can do it. Even we—in the sunsetting generation—know that, and we are counting on you to get it done.

References

Atchley D. Patient-physician communication. *In* Reynolds R, Stone J (Eds): On Doctoring. New York, NY, Simon and Schuster, 1991, pp 101–104

Augros R, Stanciu G. The New Biology: Discovering the Wisdom of Nature. Boston, Mass, Random House, 1987

Beaulieu J. Music and Sound in the Healing Arts. Barrytown, NY, Station Hill Press, 1987

Bellah R, Madsen R, Sullivan WM, Swidler A, Tipton SM. Habits of the Heart: Individualism and Commitment in American Life. New York, NY, Harper & Row, 1985

Benson H, Epstein MD. The placebo effect: a neglected asset in the care of patients. JAMA 1975; 232:1225

Benson H, McCallie DP. Angina pectoris and the placebo effect. N Engl J Med; 300:1424

Bok S. Lying. New York, NY, Pantheon Books, 1978

Breslow L. A health promotion primer for the 1990s. Health Aff 1990 Summer; 9(2):6–21

Brody H. Stories of Sickness. New Haven, Conn, Yale University Press, 1987

Bulger RJ. The humanities and the arts. *In* Bulger RJ (Ed): In Search of the Modern Hippocrates. Iowa City, Iowa,University of Iowa Press, 1987, pp 222–223

Bulger RJ. Reductionist biology and population medicine—strange bedfellows or a marriage made in heaven? JAMA 1990; 264:508–509

Bulger RJ. Emerging unities of the twenty-first century: service as sacrament, emotional neutrality, and the power of the therapeutic word. Presented at the University of Illinois Centennial Celebration, June 1992, Chicago,Ill

Burgoon JK, Pfau M, Parrott R, Birk T, Coker R, Burgoon M. Relational communication, satisfaction, compliance-gaining strategies, and compliance in communication between physicians and patients. Commun Monographs 1987; 54:307–324

Callahan D. The Troubled Dream of Life: Living with Mortality. New York, NY, Simon & Schuster, 1993

Cannon WB. Voodoo death. Amer Anthropol 1942; 44:169

Cassell EJ. The nature of suffering: physical, psychological, social, and spiritual aspects. *In* Starck PL, McGovern JP (Eds): The Hidden Dimension of Illness: Human Suffering. New York, NY, National League for Nursing Press, 1992, pp 1–10

Coles R. The Call of Service—A Witness to Idealism. Boston, Mass, Houghton Mifflin, 1993

Cousins N. Anatomy of an Illness. New York, NY, Bantam Books, 1979

Darley JM, Batson CD. From Jerusalem to Jericho: a study of situational and dispositional variables in helping behavior. J Pers Soc Psychol 1973; 27:100–108

Delbruck M. Mind from Matter? An Essay on Evolutionary Epistemology. Palo Alto, Calif, Blackwell Scientific, 1986

Eisenberg L. Science in medicine: too much or too little or too limited in scope? (background paper). *In* White KL (Ed): The Task of Medicine—Dialogue at Wickenburg. Menlo Park, Calif, The Henry J. Kaiser Family Foundation, 1988, pp 190–217

Engel GL. Sudden and rapid death during psychological stress: Folklore or folk wisdom? Ann Int Med 1971; 74:711

Engel GL. How much longer must medicine's science be bound by a seventeenth century world view? *In* White KL (Ed): The Task of Medicine—Dialogue at Wickenburg. Menlo Park, Calif, The Henry J. Kaiser Family Foundation, 1988, pp 113–136

Evans JR. The "health of the public" approach to medical education. Acad Med 1992; 67:719–723

Fee E. Disease and Discovery: A History of the Johns Hopkins School of Hygiene and Public Health 1916–1939. Baltimore, Md, Johns Hopkins University Press, 1988

Fletcher C, Freeling P. Talking and Listening to Patients: A Modern Approach. London, England, Nuffield Provincial Hospitals Trust, 1988

Fortunato JE. AIDS—The Spiritual Dilemma. New York, NY, Harper & Row, 1987

Gallimore RG, Turner JL. Contemporary studies of placebo phenomena. *In* Jarvik ME (Ed): Psychopharmacology in the Practice of Medicine. New York, NY, Appleton-Century-Crofts, 1977, p 47

Gemson DH, Elinson J. Prevention in primary care: variability in physician practice patterns in New York City. Amer J Prev Med 1986; 2: 226–234

Havens L. Making Contact: Uses of Language in Psychotherapy. Cambridge, Mass, Harvard University Press, 1986

Heitman E. The influence of values and culture in responses to suffering. *In* Starck PL, McGovern JP (Eds): The Hidden Dimension of Illness: Human Suffering. New York, NY, National League for Nursing Press, 1992, pp 81–103

Henry RC, Ogle KS, Snellman LA. Preventive medicine: physician practices, beliefs, and perceived barriers for implementation. Fam Med 1987; 19:100–113

Iglehart JK. Perspectives of an errant economist: a conversation with Tom Schelling. Health Aff 1990 Summer; 9(2):109-121

Inglefinger FJ. Medicine: meritorious or meretricious? Science 1978; 200:942

Institute of Medicine. Behavioral Influences on the Endocrine and Immune Systems. Washington, D.C., National Academy Press, 1989

Institute of Medicine. The Future of Public Health. Washington, D.C., National Academy Press, 1988

Johns MB, Hovell MF, Ganiats T, Peddecord KM, Agras WS. Primary care and health promotion: a model for preventive medicine. Am J Prev Med 1987; 6:346–358

Kennell J, Klaus M, McGrath S, Robertson S, Hinkley C. Continuous emotional support during labor in a US hospital. JAMA 1991; 265:2197–2201

Kiecolt-Glaser JK, Glaser R. Psychological influences on immunity. Psychosomatics 1986; 27:621–624

Kleinman A. The Illness Narratives: Suffering, Healing & the Human Condition. New York, NY, Basic Books, 1988

Kübler-Ross E. On Death and Dying. New York, NY, Macmillan, 1969

Kuhn TS. The Structure of Scientific Revolutions (3rd Ed). Chicago, Ill, University of Chicago Press, 1996

Lain Entralgo P. The Therapy of the Word in Classical Antiquity. New Haven, Conn, Yale University Press, 1970

Lawrence RS. The role of physicians in promoting health. Health Aff 1990 Summer; 9(2):122–132

Leversee JH: A view from general practice. *In* Bulger RJ (Ed): Hippocrates Revisited. New York, NY, Medcom, 1973, pp 93–100

Majno G. The lost secret of ancient medicine. *In* Bulger RJ (Ed): In Search of the Modern Hippocrates. Iowa City, Iowa, University of Iowa Press, 1987, pp 146–155

Marcel G. Man Against Mass Society. Chicago, Ill, Henry Regnery Company, 1962

May WF. The Patient's Ordeal. Bloomington, Ind, Indiana University Press, 1991

May WF. The Physician's Covenant: Images of the Healer in Medical Ethics. Philadelphia, Penn, Westminster Press, 1983

McDonnell TP. Thomas Merton Reader. Garden City, NY, Image Books, 1974

Mechanic D. Changing medical organization and the erosion of trust. Milbank Q 1996; 74:171–189

Milton GW. Self-willed death or the bone-pointing syndrome. Lancet 1973; 1:1435

The art of healing. Mod Healthc 1992; December 21–28:56

Mullan F. Vital Signs: A Young Doctor's Struggle with Cancer. New York, NY, Farrar, Straus, Giroux, 1975

Nuland SB. How We Die: Reflections on Life's Final Chapter. New York, NY, Knopf, 1994

Odegaard CE. Dear Doctor. Menlo Park, Calif, The Henry J. Kaiser Family Foundation, 1986

Pellegrino ED. Toward an expanded medical ethics. The Hippocratic ethic revisited. *In* Bulger RJ (Ed): Hippocrates Revisited, New York, NY, Medcom, 1973, pp 133–147

Pels RJ, Bor DH, Lawrence RS. Decision making for introducing clinical preventive services. Ann Rev Public Health 1989; 10:359–379

Pert CB, Ruff MR, Weber RJ, Herkenham M. Neuropeptides and their receptors: a psychosomatic network. J Immunol 1985; 135(suppl):820

Quill TE. Death and Dignity: Making Choices and Taking Charge. New York, NY, WW Norton, 1992

Reynolds SR, Stone J (Eds). On Doctoring. New York, NY, Simon and Schuster, 1991

Seldin D. The boundaries of medicine. Trans Assoc Am Physicians 1981; 97:75–84

Shapiro AK. Factors contributing to the placebo effect: their implications for psychotherapy. Am J Psychother 1961; 18:73

Shapiro AK. Placebo effects in psychotherapy and psychoanalysis. J Clin Pharmacol 1970; 10:73

Siegel BS. Love, Medicine, and Miracles. New York, NY, Harper & Row, 1986

Spiro HM. Placebos, patients, and physicians. *In* Bulger RJ (Ed): In Search of the Modern Hippocrates. Iowa City, Iowa, University of Iowa Press, 1987, pp 174–182

Starck PL, McGovern JP (Eds). The Hidden Dimension of Illness: Human Suffering. New York, NY, National League for Nursing Press, 1992

Starr P. The Social Transformation of American Medicine. New York, NY, Basic Books, 1982

Thomas L. House calls. *In* Reynolds R, Stone J (Eds): On Doctoring, New York, NY, Simon & Schuster, 1991, pp 203–214

Thompson T. The Wizard of Prozac. The Washington Post, November 21, 1993: p F1.

Tumulty PA. What is a clinician and what does he do? *In* Reynolds R, Stone J (Eds): On Doctoring. New York, NY, Simon and Schuster, 1991, 188–195

Turner JA, Deyo RA, Loeser JD, Von Korff M, Fordyce WE. The importance of placebo effects in pain treatment and research. JAMA 1994; 271:1609–1614

Ulrich RS. View through a window may influence recovery from surgery. Science 1984; 224:420–421

Vander Woude JC. The Caregiver as a patient. *In* Van Eys J, McGovern JP (Eds): The Doctor as a Person. Springfield, Ill, Charles C Thomas, 1988, 119–126

Vieth RF. Holy Power—Human Pain. Bloomington, Ind, Meyer Stone, 1988

Wechsler H, Levine S, Idelson RK, Rohman M, Taylor JO. The physician's role in health promotion—a survey of primary care practitioners. New Engl J Med 1983; 308:97–100

White KL. The Task of Medicine. Menlo Park, Calif, The Henry J. Kaiser Family Foundation, 1988

White KL, Connelly JE (Eds). The Medical School's Mission and the Population's Health. New York, NY, Springer-Verlag, 1992

Wolf S. Effects of suggestion and conditioning on the action of chemical agents in human subjects: the pharmacology of placebos. J Clin Invest 1950; 29:100

Wolf S, Pinsky MA. Effects of placebo administration and occurrence of toxic reactions. JAMA 1954; 155:339

Zinn WM. Transference phenomena in medical practice: being whom the patient needs. Ann Int Med 1990; 113:293–296

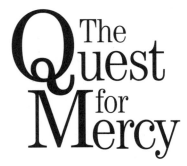

The Quest for Mercy

The forgotten ingredient in health care reform

By Roger J. Bulger, M.D.

Dear Reader,

The Quest for Mercy is a book that touches everyone—from physicians, to patients, to policymakers. It is a book about sickness and healing, hope and despair, oaths and relationships. Dr. Bulger writes about managed care with authority and passion.

The Quest for Mercy is an invaluable resource for medical students, colleagues and administrators. It will become a classic that you will want to share.

Linda Hawes Clever, M.D.
Editor, *The Western Journal of Medicine*

- -

Order Your Copies Now!

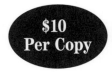

$10 Per Copy

I would like to order_____copy(ies) of **The Quest for Mercy** @ $10.00 each.*

Name _____

Institution _____

Address _____

City/State/Zip_____

Country _____

❑ Check enclosed $_____   Please charge my ❑ VISA ❑ MASTERCARD

   (*Payment must accompany order. Make check payable to:* Carden Jennings Publishing Co., Ltd.)

Account _____Expiration _____

Signature _____

MAIL TO: Carden Jennings Publishing Co., Ltd.
   1224 West Main Street, Suite 200
   Charlottesville, Virginia 22903-2858
   (804) 979-4913 • Fax: (804) 979-4025

*Note: USA/Canada postage and handling included; all other countries please add US $6.00 Air Printed Matter postage. Please add Virginia and local sales tax where applicable. Quantities of 10 or more are $6.00 each, plus shipping and handling.